Curzon's India: Networks of Colonial Governance, 1899–1905

Curzon's India: Networks of Colonial Governance, 1899–1905

Dhara Anjaria

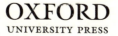
OXFORD
UNIVERSITY PRESS

OXFORD
UNIVERSITY PRESS

Oxford University Press is a department of the University of Oxford.
It furthers the University's objective of excellence in research, scholarship,
and education by publishing worldwide in

Oxford New York

Auckland Cape Town Dar es Salaam Hong Kong Karachi
Kuala Lumpur Madrid Melbourne Mexico City Nairobi
New Delhi Shanghai Taipei Toronto

With offices in

Argentina Austria Brazil Chile Czech Republic France Greece
Guatemala Hungary Italy Japan Poland Portugal Singapore
South Korea Switzerland Turkey Ukraine Vietnam

Oxford is a registered trademark of Oxford University Press
in the UK and in certain other countries

Published in Pakistan by Oxford University Press

© Oxford University Press 2014

ISBN 978-0-19-906998-9

Typeset in Adobe Garamond Pro
Printed in Pakistan by
The Times Press (Pvt) Ltd., Karachi.
Published by
Ameena Saiyid, Oxford University Press
No. 38, Sector 15, Korangi Industrial Area, PO Box 8214,
Karachi-74900, Pakistan.

Contents

Foreword

This book is a revised version of my doctoral thesis, and many people have contributed to its transformation from a thesis to a monograph.

Prof Francis Robinson and Dr Sarah Ansari of Royal Holloway College always believed in the project, even during the times I did not believe in it myself. So also, Ameena Saiyid, Managing Director of Oxford University Press Pakistan, and her team have been extremely supportive.

I should also like to thank the British Library, the National Archives at Kew, the Bodleian Library, the Library of the School of Oriental and African Studies, the Bedford Library at Royal Holloway College, the School of Slavonic and East European Studies' Library at University College London, the Coventry University Library, and also the various London Council libraries.

Research for this book was made possible by generous grants from the Sir John Plumb Charitable Trust, Cambridge, and the Indian Council of Historical Research, New Delhi. My father, Dushyant Anjaria, also supported the writing of the book through all the years it took to complete.

My thanks also to Srinivas Anirudh, who insisted that I submit the manuscript for publication. Paul and Gayle Jentz provided much needed emotional support during the writing of this book. Atul Negandhi, as always, was there when I needed him.

Dhara Anjaria
2013

1

The Viceroy's Aids to Power

George Curzon was Viceroy of India from 1899–1905, a post to which he was appointed because of his brilliance and resigned because of his intransigence and political naiveté. Curzon can be very conveniently slotted into very many interlocking sections of what Mary Fulbrook calls 'historical units of analysis'.

The Conservative Viceroy with a passion for strong control of his administration, the aristocratic Victorian globe-trotter, the Imperialist (for both his detractors and admirers), partly because of his well-defined ideological and societal placement, Curzon's Viceroyalty has attained legendary status as being symbolic of the operation and functioning of the British in India, and also as being expressive of the ideal of the same.

Curzon of Kedleston was born in Derbyshire in 1859.[1] A consciously, if sincerely, nurtured interest in parliamentary politics, so suited to a person of his birth in Victorian Britain, coupled with a passion for the imperial ideal and the foreign policy that forged it, sustained and furthered the interest in India which was crystallised when he heard Sir James Fitzjames Stephen address an Etonian audience in 1876. This was exceptional in that contemporary parliamentary front-benchers did not usually become outstanding career colonial administrators, and vice-versa. Curzon's Viceroyalty is an illustration of the difficulties of reconciling the two, both in the Viceroy's own persona and in the area of administrative coordination. His Conservative political career and the Viceregal office did not always sit easily with each other; the clashes between the two form a substantial part of this book.

As a person, Curzon was devoted to the puritan work ethic. In this he epitomised the Victorian worship of self-discipline.[2] His assessment of the Viceregal office was that it was a project 'calling for great knowledge of the country, administrative experience, unflagging energy, and almost imperious power.'[3] His preparations for Viceregal office, which took the form of travels (and resulting monographs) around the conglomeration of states and empires that ringed British India, have been too well-chronicled by all his biographers to be reproduced here yet again. He came to the office in 1898, succeeding the Earl of Elgin, and continuing the long tradition of Conservative Etonian Viceroys who had also been the pupils of Balliol master Benjamin Jowett. While his extensive knowledge of the Indian Empire was concentrated in foreign affairs and diplomatic policy, his stated aim when he took over the Viceroyalty was to spruce up and streamline Indian administration, and this was exactly what he effected, while simultaneously clarifying border policies.

Here is Curzon in 1903, the noon-tide of his Viceroyalty, writing to his Prime Minister, A.J. Balfour, with a request that his term be extended so that he could stay on and see his programme of reforms through to successful execution. In justification, he lists the achievements of his Viceroyalty thus far, and it serves as an excellent summation of his time in India, much more concise and accurate than those put forward by any of his biographers:

> The number of things that I have originated . . . is almost terrifying. . . . It is a commonplace that I have undertaken a work of reform in India in almost every branch of the administration such as has not been attempted at any period during the past half-century. . . . The new Frontier Province is working smoothly and well, and the new frontier policy is supplying cohesion and consistency to our relations with the tribes. My endeavour to stimulate the energy as well as the loyalty of the Indian Princes, and to make working bees of them in the Imperial hive . . . is everywhere bearing fruit (as their contented and happy participation in the Delhi Durbar showed); the Imperial Cadet Corps is already an assured success . . . I have settled the Berar question with the Nizam of Hyderabad . . . I have pretty well covered the whole of the native states in my tours, undertaken with the deliberate

object of bringing the head of the administration into personal contact with the Chiefs. . . .

[In] the field of internal policy and administration. . . . The new Currency Policy has had nearly four years of successful working, and the stability of Exchange seems to be satisfactorily assured. For the first time in Indian history our railways have . . . presented . . . a continuous and increasing surplus. Laws to prevent the alienation of land and the indebtedness of landholders have been passed in the Punjab and Bombay, and will shortly be passed in the United Provinces. We have dealt by legislation with the principal labour questions that I found unsettled. The growing Coal-mining industry and the Coolie labour in Assam have thus been regulated by statute. Trade and industry are on the upward gradient. Steel and ironworks are springing into existence. Outside capital and private enterprise are being attracted to our shores . . . I hope to announce to India the first great relief of taxation that it will have enjoyed for 20 years. Our Plague policy and our Famine policy have been finally evolved and . . . have taken a definite and accepted form. Agriculture, Education, Scientific research, Archaeology, which I found to be nobody's children, have all been systematised . . . and the work that is now being accomplished throughout India for the preservation, repair or restoration of ancient monuments . . . will probably be remembered long after other things are forgotten. The new rules for secretariat management, and for the reduction of reports and official writing, are in working order, and are not likely to be ignored. The Leave Rules, with their pernicious results in the frequency of official transfers, have been reformed. The Land Revenue Policy of Government . . . has been exhaustively analysed and explained in a state paper of importance; reforms have been introduced in its administration, and the principles of future working have been authoritatively laid down. The Telegraphic rates to Europe have been reduced; our sugar industry has been protected by countervailing duties against foreign bounties. . . . These are some of the things that have been done, and for which some finality or stability may perhaps be claimed.[4]

This was in 1903. Some of the most important reforms were yet to come. Among these were the irrigation reforms, the police reforms, which are widely endorsed as having been one of Curzon's most enduring reforms, and which, as he said, 'deal[t] with a subject more closely affecting the everyday life and happiness of the millions than any other aspect of administration,'[5] and the University Education Bill, as also a further consolidation of foreign policy on the Afghan frontier, and the most controversial of all—the 'Partition' of Bengal.

Yet this impressive track record did not prevent the Home Government accepting his resignation with alacrity after he failed to convince them that he, not Kitchener, was right about the issue of military reform in India. This raises questions as to the actual potency of this undoubtedly brilliant and committed Viceroy. This, then, is the line of enquiry this work follows, and the main question that it seeks to answer. *Curzon and the Limits of Viceregal Power: India, 1899-1905,* therefore, seeks to understand 'how key individuals were able to shape, constrain and transform the field of historical forces in which they operated,'[6] and, reflectively, had their own actions shaped, constrained, and transformed by these forces. It explores the power balances in the Viceroy's administrative relations with various sectors and persons within the British Government of India and those who moved on its fringes or were co-opted into its hegemonic framework. The main thrust of the work is towards examining the kind of relationships Curzon had with the different sectors of the British Government of India—and whether his biographers, even the most sympathetic of them, were right when they claimed that his lack of inter-personal skills ruined his Indian tenure, or, more precisely, whether the contention that he lacked inter-personal skills holds true at all.

Superficially, there appears to be no need to debate as to whether Curzon exercised power and influence in India, whatever negotiations he might have been compelled to make with London. He was, after all, the head of the administration, and could be assumed to be invested with a certain amount of *ex-officio* power. But just as studies of his predecessor underscore Elgin's inability to make an impact upon the administration of India, it follows that the holding of office does not necessarily translate into the ability to utilise the powers afforded by that office. Did Curzon utilise his? More pertinently, was he able to?

Contested power and authority reveal themselves through friction in working relationships; when people recognise and accept their respective places in a known hierarchy, they tend to conform to the *status quo*. Curzon's assumption of the Viceroyalty caused considerable tumult within the established patterns of deference in the Indian administration; the civil servants found that bureaucratic administration, formerly their sole preserve, was being minutely examined and modified by the Viceroy; the Secretary of State was confronted (though not without some inkling of what was to come) with a Viceroy who staked out a separate identity for India, the Indians found a zealous champion for their rights, who was yet more unwilling than most to accord *them* a measure of administrative autonomy for these functionaries, Curzon upset their boundaries of authority. But to what extent, if at all, did they resist or comply with what they could potentially view as uncalled-for infringement upon their spheres?

The question of how much power was exercised by proconsuls in general has been explored by Mark Francis.[7] Zoe Laidlaw[8] has considered this issue further by looking at the networks which helped colonial administrators gain influence both in their own colonies and with the government in London. Laidlaw notes how being part of a network, i.e., knowing people, helped colonial administrators gain access to the right places for achieving their objectives. How relevant is this argument in the case of Curzon, a man who biographers allege lost out precisely because of the pressures and expectations old connections placed on official relationships? While there has not been much cross-pollination between works dealing with Imperial history and scholars working on Curzon in India, especially in terms of methodology—the extant work on Curzon in India being largely empiricist. Curzon's early biographer, Kenneth Rose, takes a step towards examining the effect of state politics carried on by a small elite circle upon the social relations of the persons concerned.[9] Rose analyses how these same social networks functioned as channelling factors and delineated Curzon's political fortunes, especially his Viceregal relationship with Whitehall. He also posits the social and cultural background of the age as a strong influential factor in the way Curzon's life unfolded. Rose's work, however, stops short of actually spelling out the effect Curzon's personal relationships with Cabinet members had on their reception of his plans as Viceroy, and is also confined to Home politics. This book is then a logical furtherance and development of Rose's work, expanding upon this theme, while adding a colonial dimension to it, as well as reversing Rose's methodology, and looking at the effect social relations had upon the execution of state politics.

Curzon's principal biographers tend to deliver a uniform verdict when it comes to assessing his time in India. Penderel Moon notes that with Curzon as Governor General, the 'Government of India became for a while very nearly an autocracy . . . [but] the outcome of his seven years of office was politically not at all what he intended.'[10] S. Gopal, who has produced some of the most insightful Indian scholarship on Curzon, explains this by stating that 'the essence of [successful administration] is an easy command of men, and of this Curzon was incapable.'[11] Others have theorised that Curzon was disinclined to teamwork rather than being incapable of it. David Gilmour observes that, 'Curzon never tried to delegate,'[12] and also that he did not listen, or rather, engage with people in a position to advise him about anything.[13] While Gilmour does not assess Curzon's ability to convince people in India, this point is not taken up by David Dilks,[14] either, whose sympathetic biography does not really engage with Curzon's dealings with his Indian colleagues in detail. Thus the negotiations, the deliberations and the ups and downs that Curzon experienced in his efforts to get Mackworth Young, Antony MacDonnell, Arthur Havelock, Lord Ampthill, Lords Sandhurst and Northcote to agree to his reforms, go un-explored. This may be, in part, due to the assumption that because these functionaries were anyway Curzon's subordinates, how they interacted with him would not affect him politically, but, as Peter King has shown, a perceived slight to any individual could be crucial in turning that person against the Viceroy.[15]

These blanket statements, and often the particular historiographic approach adopted, for example, biographical narratives in general leave little room for in-depth analysis or the application of inter-disciplinary concepts to seven years of an action-packed life, or the web of interpersonal relations, given that their focus is on the one man mean that neither Curzon's team-building skills, nor his skills at political manipulation, have been explored, because the assumption is that he did not listen to anyone's opinions (or opposition), which of course precludes the possibility of arguing with, and persuading, or coercing, them into seeing his side of the matter.

In fact there are many questions relating to the level of authority exercised by Curzon in India that have either not been explored in detail, or not explored from a particular angle, or overlooked by scholars, the most glaring omission being that of Curzon's relationship with Lord Ampthill, Governor of Madras 1900–1906 and Curzon's locum in 1904.

The question of how Curzon engaged with, and persuaded (or not) people to support the legislation he pushed through has also not been explored. It is true that his contretemps with the India Council over its refusal to accede to some of his requests has been cited as proof of his intractability and inability to persuade through negotiation, but this analysis has never been extended to include his provincial governors, the Indian Civil Service, and the Indians. Also unexplored is the degree to which, if at all, his influence over his colleagues waxed and waned throughout his term in office; if such were the case, it would suggest that his influence throughout his Viceroyalty was not uniform, rather subjective and dependent on time and place, and the person he was dealing with.

There are assumptions about Curzon in India, too, germane to the question of his authority and influence, which have gained popular currency even when there is a case for refuting them through historical evidence, a prime example being the popular contention that he was simultaneously ineffectual and autocratic, and that he did not have the influence, nor leave the legacy, he sought, precisely because of his autocracy. This assumption, along with Curzon's well-known penchant for doing everything himself, has led to a tacit understanding among scholars of Empire that Curzon was not a team player. Winston Churchill, a contemporary who observed Curzon in India, states that the ultimate transience of Curzon's legacy lay in the fact that he could never, because of his lack of knowledge of handling men, found a dedicated band of followers.[16] This seemingly authoritative endorsement from someone famed for his ability to strike a chord with everyone he came into contact with has only served to confirm the professional historian's view that Curzon had no people skills.

This book attempts to address, and refute, this contention as well, examining the issues touched upon above by using Curzon's relationship with various significant components of the then political landscape of the Government of India, devoting a chapter to each of the significant areas where Curzon's impact needs further elucidation. It deliberately explores these questions in the context of Curzon's domestic, or internal, administration, because this was the area he was least knowledgeable about when he assumed office, and also the area where current and former Indian administrators, and of course the Indians themselves, could pose, by virtue of their long experience, the strongest challenge to his primacy. He was more or less the recognised authority on the Frontier so his political capital wouldn't suffer in the event he was unable to carry his officers and governors with him insofar as Frontier Policy was concerned—and in fact this was indeed the case.

Hence, this book is also a refutation of some of the contentions laid out by Curzon's principal biographers: Kenneth Rose, David Dilks, S. Gopal, and David Gilmour, all of whom gain legitimacy because their conclusions are based on readings of the personal papers of the principal actors; this book counters their contentions about Curzon's poor personnel management skills limiting his clout using largely the same sources. Most biographies and studies of Curzon in India are largely the product of empiricist research, but for that method—'scientific history, based on the rigorous investigation of primary sources'[17]—to be effective, must look at the sources in their totality. This has not happened where Curzon was concerned.

The history of British India from Clive to Curzon finds a glory in the fact of a coterie of traders single-handedly conquering an entire subcontinent; and Curzon's claim that if one wanted a thing well-done, it was best to do it oneself, is quoted by old India hands not without a sense of the romance of its misguided valour; but Plassey was won in conjunction, and with the support, of what may best be described as a collaborator. Similarly, Curzon was aided by a host of factors which helped him exercise his *ex-officio* power. This chapter will examine factors that helped him wield the kind of influence he wanted to over the administration of India and the people responsible for assenting the policies of the Government of India.

Nigel Nicolson notes that Curzon started out with very many advantages as compared to other recent incumbents of the Viceregal chair: 'the respect of the House of Commons, his intimate friendship with leading men in Government and Opposition, their conviction that only Curzon was capable of reforming Indian administration from top to bottom.'[18] While the precise advantages may be subject to question, and indeed have been refuted by other research, there is no denying that Curzon benefited vastly from a set of factors which colluded to ensure he ran the Government of India as much his own way as possible. Some of these factors helped him clinch his appointment and launch out smoothly; some came to light and developed over the course of his term. The very fact of his succeeding the incumbents he did ensured that he was viewed as a welcome change. His predecessors counted among themselves the languid Elgin, of whom it was said that he should never have left his Scottish estate, Lansdowne, not really very outstanding, and Lytton, whose foreign policy was largely dominated by Salisbury in London. Given this, a Viceroy with boundless zeal, who had already circumnavigated the globe and produced a pile of authoritative volumes on geo-politics out of it, was viewed with a sense of relief that India, in India, would have the benefit of an interested administrator.

Curzon's worldview was defined by sets of attributes he possessed, by ideologies he adhered to, by the people and ideas he came into contact with. For instance, it is safe to assume that Curzon's righteous and rigidly mapped out views about the running of the administration were congruent with a 'less-the-better' approach towards uninformed opposition. He candidly professed that he knew more about the problems of India than anyone else, by virtue of having expended his adult life studying them, and this in fact was one factor that earned him the right to do what he liked, largely, as regards governing the country. A large part of Curzon's authority was, in fact, derived from his expert knowledge of Asian affairs. To start with, this was the factor which, overriding all other concerns, was the one which ensured that Curzon was appointed as Viceroy. In fact, it may be said that it was solely on the strength of this one virtue that he applied for, and was granted, the Viceregal office, and this was no mean achievement considering that the trend then was towards proconsuls who knew little about India and were much too intimidated to learn more. Curzon's knowledge gave him an edge. As noted in Chapter Four, it was this which enabled him to override the objections of Mackworth Young, Governor of Punjab, when carving out the NWFP (North-West Frontier Province) from that province.

This section, drawing upon the events analysed in the core chapters, examines what factors enabled Curzon to exercise as much power and authority as he liked, unfettered and unhampered. It lists the people and phenomena responsible for helping, or supporting him, push through and execute legislation, planning and pronouncements that tallied with his self-styled plan for governing the Indian Empire. Two factors need to be gauged: the lack of opposition he was confronted with, and the level of support he was given, each of which would have very different implications on the outcome of his actions, even though they might have enabled the same thing: letting Curzon have his way. As Dowding states, 'political power is qualified by the fact that the people who exercise it make, [consciously], the decisions they do after weighing the underlying factors. It is a rational exercise.' From this, one may infer that it is not the individual's sole and unfettered will which he himself, even, takes into account when making political decisions.

What, then, were the well-springs of support that Curzon drew upon? There are two kinds of resources of power, 'bases of resources that make possible its exercise,'[19] and 'resources [the individual] brings to the power relation that enable him to exercise power.'[20] People could be classified as the former, but unless the individual wishing to exercise power makes some effort to co-opt them, they would remain an unutilised resource. Thus, ultimately, it is the individual's own will-to-power that is crucial in determining, at the very least, his efforts to exercise authority. Thus, there are factors intrinsic to the individual's mental makeup, factors circumstantial to his setting, and factors totally extrinsic, for example, other people, who may have their own, often conflicting, self-interests in aiding the individual who seeks to attain power. This chapter divides Curzon's 'resources of power' into two main categories: the people and the circumstantial.

Superficially, it would not appear that people could be an asset to Curzon in his quest for power and authority, as it has been assumed by even his admirers that 'a Curzon kindergarten . . . a band of younger men who gave him total allegiance and implemented his principles and policies with full understanding . . . was inconceivable.'[21] But, as shall be demonstrated below, this was in fact what happened. Curzon may have tossed away some of the advantages his prodigious skills afforded him by alienating a great many of the people who were best placed to help him maximise his impact upon Indian administration, but nevertheless, there were certain people who smoothed the path of the Viceroyalty greatly. It may in fact be said that he managed to establish close working relationships with these individuals, and while he never had the sort of informal lobby that surrounded, say, A.J. Balfour or St. John Brodrick, he did have loyal supporters across many departments of the government at home and in India. The first, and perhaps the most influential of these was George Hamilton.

George Francis Hamilton had been Secretary of State for India for three years when Curzon was appointed Viceroy, an appointment Hamilton regarded with some circumspection, given Curzon's reputation for Russophobia.[22] But the Curzon–Hamilton relationship was one of the more successful partnerships of Curzon's time in India. As Dilks notes, had Curzon agreed to have, in 1905, the investigating committee over the issue of the Military Supply Member out, the outcome would almost certainly have gone against Kitchener, because Hamilton was to have been on the committee.[23] Of course, the most important reason that Hamilton backed Curzon was because he—Curzon—could be trusted to know what was what in relation to India, and Hamilton knew this. It is noteworthy that Curzon's most significant legislation came in when Hamilton was at the India Office, but Hamilton's value did not only lie in being a more accommodating Secretary of State than Brodrick (he colluded with Curzon over leaving out Mackworth Young from the deliberations over creating the NWFP). Hamilton actively backed Curzon's measures; his actions helped deflect criticism of Curzon from others in the India Office or the Cabinet. The relationship between Curzon and Hamilton, in fact, was one of collusion, somewhat like the rapport the heads of two otherwise mutually hostile states might share. The reasons put forth by Curzon's biographers are that Hamilton agreed with many of Curzon's ideas in principle, and also that he had occupied his post long enough to assert this, and that finally, he had no incentive to prove himself against Curzon, unlike his successor and Curzon's schoolmate St. John Brodrick. But one needs to theorise about the self-incentives available to Hamilton via this support for Curzon—what did he stand to gain?

Hamilton, whatever his personal inclinations were, ultimately derived his power by being part of the machine that was the India Office. He held constitutional power over Curzon, but his own power was not autonomous; it was derived from something extrinsic to himself. In a large organization, Foucault noted, 'one doesn't have . . . a power which is wholly in the hands of one person who can exercise it alone and totally over others. It is a machine in which everyone is caught, those who exercise power just as much as those over whom it is exercised.'[24] Thus is not unreasonable to expect that the two parties might collude to protect their interests from the power that is superior to *both* of them. Hamilton, who liked to keep the peace, lived in fear of a parliamentary investigation into Indian affairs.[25] Curzon, who did not particularly care about the peace, had no such inhibitions, and unwittingly made the burden of pouring oil onto troubled waters over to Hamilton, who readily assumed it. This may have been, because, as can be evidenced from the many times Hamilton tried to reason with Curzon, while he had 'power to' over Curzon, but he did not have 'power over'[26] to make him do things Curzon was disinclined to doing. This can be attributed to historical circumstances—Hamilton's position was cramped at the India Office. Brodrick could attempt the carrot-and-stick method with Curzon (that Curzon did not take notice of it being quite another matter) because he was part of a close-knit ruling cabinet. But Hamilton was prevented by circumstances from using incentive structures. As long as Salisbury was alive and in power, Hamilton was not in a position to make a conditional incentive, given that this could be over-ridden by a directive from Salisbury, whose protégé Curzon was. Nor could he make an unconditional threat because he was ultimately subject to the censure of Godley, the permanent Under-Secretary who wielded tremendous influence. Also, as noted above, he did not have 'power over' Curzon because Curzon knew—and Hamilton knew, and admitted, that he knew more than he did about India. In this instance Curzon's prowess won out over Hamilton's. He was able to put down enough unconditional incentives—or threats—ensuring that these were successful by pre-committing himself to carrying them out (in his case this meant resignation) in the event of non-compliance to his wishes from the India Office and Whitehall.[27] All this meant that Curzon enjoyed the support of the Secretary of State, and thus had a voice in London while in India. Hamilton was, in every sense, a mediator.

Finally, Hamilton also appears to have known how to handle Godley and the delicate subject of sharing Curzon's correspondence with him. Nowhere was this more essential than where Arthur Olivier Villiers Russell, 2nd Baron Ampthill, Governor of Madras 1900–1906, was concerned.

When Curzon expostulated against the absurdity of a man of thirty-four being handed the Viceroyalty while he himself went on leave, Hamilton observed that at least Ampthill would keep up the ceremonial side of the Viceregal office very well.[28] But there was substance behind Ampthill's self-assured façade; it was not the only point where he resembled Curzon. Indeed, one of the major themes of this book is the assertion that Ampthill's backing was Curzon's major support during the intrigue ridden final months of his Viceroyalty.

Ampthill in his capacity as Lieutenant Governor of Madras has been more often utilised by historians to demonstrate the friction-laden relationship between Simla and the presidencies, but as Chapters Two, Three, and Five demonstrate, having a Governor like Ampthill greatly aided Curzon in the later stages of his Viceroyalty. It was not just over the major incidents that Ampthill supported his chief; their views on many aspects of administration tallied. This enabled the creation of a uniform characteristic of administration across India, enabling the ruling British to present a homogeneous façade before the governed. As in the case of Hamilton, it helped that Ampthill, when not considering solely the parochial interests of Madras Presidency, had much the same political views as Curzon. For instance, he was the Governor who most closely matched Curzon's attitudes towards Indians. He seems to have shared Curzon's dislike of the 'hybrid university educated mule,' stating that 'the unofficial native of the Madras Presidency, who is competent to serve on a big Commission or to pronounce opinions worth having on any big question, is practically non-existent. It is a sad fact that we have no prominent men outside the ranks of Judges, Barristers and officials.'[29] Yet he was also, as shall be seen in Chapter Three, one of the first to institute affirmative action for Indians from the depressed classes, much as Curzon strove for a humane treatment of all Indians. As an instrument for the delegation of political power, thus, Ampthill was eminently suitable for Curzon's preferred style of administration. One only wonders whether, had Ampthill instead of Sandhurst or Northcote, been Governor of Bombay, the intellectual seat of the nationalist movement, the said movement would have survived his term of office.

But it was as Acting Viceroy in 1904 that Ampthill really helped Curzon keep a hold over Indian polity, by the simple process of sticking, in the face of increasing opposition from the India Office, to Curzon's line of thought. That he did so demonstrates that Curzon exercised a certain amount of authority over Ampthill. Ampthill's acting Viceroyalty was an example of the successful delegation of power. Ampthill also helped Curzon by refusing to be taken, or to act, lightly because of the temporary nature of his term in office. The connection between power and responsibility can be said to be 'essentially negative: you can deny all responsibility by demonstrating lack of power,'[30] but Ampthill did not resort to this tactic. He did not give in to the demands of the India Office once he had decided to follow Curzon's line in administrative affairs, even though it would have been beneficial for him to do so. Ampthill goes against the accepted model seen by theorists: that it is safe to stick to one ideology because it affords protection within the group and also requires less effort than changing it.[31] He not only turned around his initial working relationship with Curzon, (which, following the best of centre-provincial tradition, started off acrimoniously), but did not return to his initial position even when explicitly encouraged by the India Office to do so. It was found by French and Synder that 'opponents who changed their opinions (as Ampthill did about Curzon) toward the leader . . . were more certain of their new opinions. Within groups there was a trend in the same direction.'[32] This latter statement is also true of Curzon's Viceroyalty: his relationship with Ampthill settled down just as his relationship with the Governor of Bombay, Northcote, blossomed. This is however in line with accepted theoretical models. The increasing degree of willing followership that Ampthill assumed in relation to Curzon can also be vindicated by the same study: 'the more the group leader is accepted by another member of the group, the more effective will be his attempts to influence this member.'[33] Ampthill, thus, is the refutation of S. Gopal's claim that Curzon never gathered any followers.

MARY LEITER

Curzon's biographers have universally noted that it was at variance with his character that he married an American, their justification for this stance being that a person so rooted in English patriarchal modes of being would prefer to source a wife from a similar background, to supplant his cementing within that sub-culture. But as other observers have pointed out, Anglo–American alliances were rather popular in the late Victorian period,[34] and Curzon, as has been demonstrated earlier, was very much in tune with contemporary social nuances; in fact he moulded himself, consciously or unconsciously, upon what he perceived an ideal young man of that age should be like, and therefore it is not uncommon that with respect to matrimony too, he should have chosen a wife in accordance with what was commonly taking place among his peers and contemporaries.

Of course, Curzon's primary motive in marrying the Chicago born Mary Leiter, it has been hypothesised—and dismissed—by Nicolson, Gilmour, and Kenneth Rose, was not social conformity, but money. This brings us to the first and most concrete way in which Curzon's marriage facilitated his having an easier time as Viceroy: financially, it enabled him to take up the Viceroyalty, which it is doubtful that he would otherwise have been able to do. As Mary's biographer observes, Levi Leiter made a marriage settlement of £140,000 and in addition granted Mary an allowance of £6000 per annum. Even after Joseph Leiter's disastrous attempt to corner the American grain market just as Curzon was taking up the Viceroyalty, Levi helped out with £3000.[35] As Kenneth Galbraith noted, the 'power of property' was extremely high in the later years of the nineteenth century. By this he meant that property—wealth in the form of cash, land, and other assets—accorded power to its possessor. Drawing upon this, it may be argued that in Curzon's case, property—his, via his wife's—was the integument that held his Viceroyalty together.[36]

Observers have also noted that Mary helped his Viceroyalty in a very politically tangible way by making efforts to reach out to official and non-official sections of the populace and the British in India, something Edwina Mountbatten was to achieve with a good deal more success forty-seven years later. She seemed more accessible than Curzon, (she was at her most effective when people sought her intercession, and not when she tried to change the course of political relations), and there probably existed a feeling that she could change his stance on certain issues, which of course, she self-admittedly could not. The perception of accessibility may have evolved simply because she was not actually vested with formal office and the distance such office instils between the office holder and the lay public. Still, even Curzon's estranged Punjab governor wrote to her seeking to normalise relations:

> you have always been very kind to me and I can't tell you how much I have valued your friendship . . . it is through no act of mine that the cessation of friendly relations between Viceregal Lodge and Barnes Court has come about. Someone has evidently carried false reports about me to H.E. the Viceroy, and he actually believes that I have 'vilified and abused' him all over Simla.[37]

The third and final way, and one for which we have Curzon's strongest admission, in which Mary helped Curzon's Viceroyalty was by being his wife, and by her way of carrying this out. If being undemanding and supportive fits rather too well into the modes of classical wifehood, it should be remembered that this was what Curzon wanted and expected from a wife and Vicereine, and possibly because he felt that this did indeed provide him with the best possible support than a wife who typed his letters, it just might have done so, mostly because of the mental solace it afforded him.

While this book does not seek to analyse Mary Leiter's role in making or breaking Curzon's political fortunes, it is worth a mention. As it was an age in which boudoir conspiracy was the norm, one has only to look at Lady Salisbury's part in the Kitchener Affair, or the concern over Margot Tennant marrying H.H. Asquith, to understand the much larger role backroom scenes played in that era—it was not what Curzon wanted, and while he always told Mary she was good for his political fortunes, he would have scorned any suggestion that she actively use her guile to help him. It is also true that Mary was seen as something of a political lightweight by Curzon's contemporaries, and how this affected his Viceroyalty will be examined later.

As noted above, people do not operate out of context to the circumstances they find themselves in, nor do the circumstances take shape autonomously. It was the unique interaction of events on the political stage, the people behind the events, and Curzon's approach to these that determined the level of influence he exercised as Viceroy. He has been criticised for his seeming attempt to run the Government of India as a one-man show, but even this attempt shaped its own impact. The qualities for which Curzon was appointed to office and how he brought these to bear upon the interactions that office required are discussed below.

EXPERT KNOWLEDGE OF ASIAN AFFAIRS

There is no direct correlation between knowledge and power, in fact, 'seen from the perspective of power, the problem of ideology or knowledge revolves around its capacity to achieve results, especially through forms of ideological incorporation or hegemony.'[38] Thus, as will be illustrated at the close of the book, Curzon's expertise can only be considered an asset insofar as it helped him convince others to follow his schemes. But, in 1899, the fact of his being a well-travelled scholar-explorer was the reason Curzon was awarded the Viceroyalty; indeed, it was the basis upon which he had begged for it. There was, in fact, no other justification for him being appointed Viceroy; his abrasiveness was well-known, there were other, better connected claimants for the post, and he had only held one major posting before this one as Undersecretary for India. But for someone whose view of the rest of Empire was that it merely constituted the 'toll-gates and the barbicans' of The Empire, India, he had prepared himself thoroughly for the Viceroyalty by inspecting every one of those edifices, as well as India itself. From 1887 to 1895, Curzon traversed Persia, the Far East, the Straits Settlements, Afghanistan, and India to study the layout of Imperial authority in relation to the Indian Empire. His writings on these remain authoritative works today. In 1898, they were considered sufficient for Salisbury to appoint someone who was otherwise just an Undersecretary for Foreign Affairs to the most important colonial posting the Empire could offer. (Not that Curzon saw it as a *colonial*, in the sense of marginal position.)

If, then, there were no murmurings apart from those of the disgruntled Punjab governor when Curzon put through the creation of the NWFP, it was because it was known he had spent years travelling on the frontier and could be expected to gauge its temper accurately. This would approximate to Max Weber's concept of 'charismatic authority', which, resting, as it does, in part, 'on devotion to the specific and exceptional sanctity, heroism or exemplary character of an individual person,'[39] would have enabled Curzon to deny the established forms of authority.[40] As Edward VII commented, 'the reason Curzon is making so good a Viceroy is that beside his great personal ability he has personal knowledge of the country.'[41]

Coupled with his knowledge, Curzon brought a good deal of enthusiasm to the task of over-hauling the administration. This inspired devotion for reform made him drag out and finish long-standing and complex projects. He did not confine his knowledge to the realms of pedagogy, as Denzil Ibbetson, one of the most prominent administrators of the late nineteenth century, observed:

> It has not only been a pleasure to work under Your Excellency. It has also been an education. Your splendid energy, your, if possible, still more splendid

courage and confidence in the right, your single-minded devotion to the
good of India and her people, and your wonderful power of mastering every
detail while never losing sight of broad principles and the end in view, have
made you the most stimulating chief conceivable. . . . I decline to
contemplate the event of your not returning to us. There is so much still to
be done: and it is such a stimulus to work, to feel assured that whatever may
be decided on will be carried through with an unfaltering hand. . . .[42]

Thus Curzon, according to his officers, inspired people to work with his
own work ethic and determination to do good. Even his detractors
conceded that his fractiousness was brought about by overwork, and
were therefore inclined to overlook it. Also it led him to press his suit
with a degree of vehemence and persistence that could not be ignored—
for example the Salt Tax reduction; a lesser Viceroy might have quailed
under the rebuff, but Curzon extracted concessions.

In all this Curzon's undoubted charisma was helped along by the non-
reputations of his relatively lackadaisical predecessors, Lansdowne and
Elgin. His abilities were estimated rather more highly than they might
have been had he succeeded an outstanding Viceroy. Nor, unlike Wavell,
did he have to contend with a rising star on the horizon; with Selborne
having taken himself off for South Africa, the imminent prospect, in
1903, of having St. John Brodrick as the next Viceroy (he had just
endured a horrendous run at the War Office) ensured that Curzon
greatly went up in the estimation of British official opinion.

There were stray grumblings about Curzon's relative youth when
appointed Viceroy, but he managed to turn this fact into a celebration
of his extraordinary abilities. And once he became Viceroy, the factor
was discounted; what mattered was the fact that he was the highest
British official in India. This was the effect of the traditionally
hierarchical structure of the Raj, which enabled people to tolerate his
bossing them around; the expectation was that people would pull around
to doing what he wished. It was a matter of cohesiveness—Kipling's
great lumbering machine prompted a degree of obedience and

conformity: 'the individual [in this case individual officer] submits to the common purposes of the organization, and from this internal exercise of power comes the ability of organization to impose its will externally, i.e., being able to run India efficiently.' Thus, from strong internal organization came external power, a concept which was probably at the core of Curzon's Viceroyalty.[43] This structure, with its minute gradations of seniority, earned Curzon the default following of the ICS (Indian Civil Service). As Walter Lawrence observed, once the ICS noted his prodigious capacity for work, they grudgingly began to acknowledge his self-proclaimed extra-ordinariness.[44] This may be evidenced in Ibbetson's acknowledgement of Curzon above.

But this argument brings the reader back full circle to the previous paragraph: British India's 77 place Warrant of Precedence. If the ICS followed Curzon because of the strong culture of respecting seniority of office, and this benefited Curzon, it can also be argued, again, that he was able to command the allegiance of this pool of talent because of the prestige of his office. Colonial historians tend to dismiss the pomp, circumstance and exaggerated respect that surrounded high administrative office in Victorian times as the folly of an age that still saw deep crevasses between the rulers and the ruled, but there was more to the elephant rides than over-awing the resentful rabble.[45] That Curzon was anointed Viceroy, head of the administration, did not hurt at all. It conferred upon him that what sociologists refer to as legitimate authority, and identify as one of the most important appurtenances of power: Dahl, Wrong, Sennett, Weber all rank it, along with cash, as somewhere near the apex of an 'importance-pyramid'. And in the rigidly hierarchical environment of British India, it probably can be placed higher than cash or material assets. Thus, the prestige accorded to the office of Viceroy was not merely constitutional or ceremonial. The fact of being Viceroy endowed Curzon with the powers to be a leader, to exercise his authority over other people in India, who were made necessarily, and legally, subordinate to him. Legitimate authority is in fact one of the major resources of power, and is mostly always utilised in full.[46] Curzon achieved this not only by highlighting the fact that he was Viceroy, but, where this placed him lower than a colleague in official hierarchy—as in his dealings with the Secretary of State—he always emphasised how fortunate the office was to have so capable and able an incumbent as himself. It enabled him, in theory, to cut down all opposition even if the opposition could be held equally, if not more so, well-informed on a given subject—obviously 'in an ongoing game, a piece like the Queen would start in a more privileged position than a pawn, simply because the extant rules . . . enable her to begin the sequence with more potential moves to make.'[47] Very simply, Curzon could remove a bureaucrat from his post if he disagreed with him as a matter of course; the same course of action was not open to the bureaucrat.

The Viceregal office endowed Curzon with the authority to do the things he wanted to; without the benefit of the Viceregal chair, his proclamations on India would have remained those of a pamphleteering politician, to be received with a degree of annoyance by the establishment, which, indeed, was the case after his resignation in 1905. Thus, his knowledge and expertise were legitimised *ex-officio*. The Viceregal office, therefore, may also be said to approximate to Max Weber's concept of 'traditional authority—where obedience is owed to the person of the chief who occupies the traditionally sanctioned position of authority. . . .'[48] This was what enabled indifferent Viceroys serve out their terms without any trouble; it was also the cloak behind which an over-zealous Viceroy might mask his zeal and yet be implicitly obeyed. Curzon's position was stronger while backed by Hamilton, because that was an indication that his actions were endorsed by his constitutional superiors in London, 'the perception of illegitimacy would eventually erode the strength seen in an authority.'[49] It also meant that there was one less avenue of complaint left open to anyone disgruntled with Curzon's policies. Thus, this one fact of Curzon's official existence in India incorporated many levels and forms of authority and power.

GROWING TREND TOWARDS CENTRALIZATION

Curzon's detractors may not have liked his tendency to attempt a concentration of the reins of administration in his hand, and it was this battle over centralization that soured a good many relations (Curzon–Havelock and Curzon–Whitehall, for example) but it meant that more decisions were taken at the centre with a pan-Indian impact in mind, as opposed to becoming purely local concerns. Obviously this let Curzon exercise his love for detail. It also ensured that the governors became rather more answerable to him. He wanted collaboration and this was one way of ensuring that it was achieved. It was not possible for a Presidency Governor under Curzon to assume the sort of independence exercised by Bartle Frere and Mountstuart Elphinstone; the governors' symbolic as well as real power diminished as the *Viceroy's* stature increased correspondingly. Also, that period marked a growing centralization towards London, which shows that the India Office was not opposed to the concept of centralization per se. What they did object to was it being exercised by someone who was not doing it their way.

Centralization per se has many benefits: it means a 'good chance of achieving and maintaining concentrations of resources, speed and consistency of decision-making, high visibility and orientation for their clients looking for service.'[50]

INDIAN PUBLIC OPINION

Up until the disastrous Calcutta Convocation speech and the Partition of Bengal (1905), and even censure of this last measure was not universal among Indians, Curzon's measures were very well received by most sections of the Indian press. Such accolades helped him carry off stuff without fear of Indian reprisals, and also bolstered his conviction that he was going the right way about ensuring the contentment of the governed. In this his crusade against racial discrimination helped. As will be explored in Chapter Six, Indian public opinion across India was extremely favourable, right up until the time of the Partition of Bengal.

In those days, Indian public opinion could hardly be said to be based on common nationalistic grounds, and Anglophone public opinion largely expressed itself through the press, letters and representations made to the Viceroy and other officials. Even Curzon's uncompromising opposition to Indian self-representation had a silver lining: it had the effect of keeping them quiet, as according to C. Friedrich's rule of anticipated reactions, people will not press for demands if they feel they will not get anywhere.[51]

Indian approbation and Curzon were cyclical. It must be remembered that, in 1899, the nascent nationalist movement was not necessarily anti-British, but more concerned with securing equalitarian treatment under British rule. If, then, they got a Viceroy who kept the scales even, it fulfilled their expectations from British rule. A large section of the Indian press reflected the interests of the many sections of the populace who were rather more concerned about the impact government legislation might have on their lifestyles, as opposed to fighting for a concept they did not yet feel had reached them, i.e., Indian nationalism. This is most starkly illustrated in the case of the Punjab Land Alienation Act; while the Congress campaigned against it, Punjab's local Indian press overwhelmingly supported it, and those papers that did oppose it opposed specific terms that they felt might inadvertently hinder them in carrying out their business.

This chapter, then, has set out the advantages which Curzon enjoyed as he began his term. He started off with a formidable battery of the tangibles and intangibles of power. When he landed in Bombay on 30 December 1898, however, he landed in enemy territory. The Governor of Bombay, Lord Sandhurst, and his counterpart in Madras, Sir Arthur Elibank Havelock, did not subscribe to the view that they should subordinate themselves, or their provinces, to his authority at all. This rather tended to render irrelevant the many ways by which exercising that authority was made easy for Curzon. While Chapter Three explores Curzon's relationship with the part of *British* India that sought autonomy as an 'ancient privilege', and the lobbying for whose Lieutenant

Governorships went on, if at all, in London and not amongst the top brass of India's civil service: the Presidencies of Madras and Bombay, the next chapter looks at the entities they appealed to in the battle for autonomy from Simla, Curzon's constitutional superiors, the India Office.

Notes

1. The Curzons were of Norman descent and had come over with William the Conqueror. They had held the estate of Kedleston in Derbyshire for 800 years when George was born. While Kedleston Hall was architecturally renowned, the estate was by no means as prosperous as those held by many of Curzon's contemporaries. The lack of belonging to the highest echelons of titled Victorian society may have spurred Curzon on to even greater eminence than he might otherwise have tried for. For a relevant assessment that links Curzon's background to his political life, see Kenneth Rose, *Curzon: A Most Superior Person*, (London: Macmillan, 1985 [1969]), pp. 1–8.
2. Iain Pears, 'The Gentleman and the Hero: Wellington and Napoleon in the Nineteenth Century', in *Leadership: Classical, Contemporary and Critical Approaches*, Keith Grint (ed.), (Oxford: Oxford University Press, 1997), p. 232.
3. Curzon to Balfour, 05 February 1903, Balfour Papers, Add. Mss 49732.
4. Curzon to Balfour, 05 February 1903, Balfour Papers, Add. Mss 49732.
5. Curzon to Balfour, 05 February 1903, Balfour Papers, Add. Mss 49732.
6. Fulbrook, *Historical Theory*, p. 78.
7. Mark Francis, *Governors & Settlers: Images of Authority in the British Colonies, 1820-60*, (Basingstoke: Macmillan, 1992).
8. Zoe Laidlaw, *Colonial Connections*, (Manchester: MUP, 2005).
9. Kenneth Rose, *Curzon: A Most Superior Person*, (London: Macmillan, 1985 [1969]).
10. Sir Penderel Moon, *The British Conquest and Dominion of India*, (London: Duckworth, 1989), p. 911.
11. S. Gopal, *British Policy in India, 1858-1905*, (Cambridge: Cambridge University Press, 1965), p. 225.
12. David Gilmour, *Curzon: Imperial Statesman*, (London: John Muray, 1994), p. 216.
13. Ibid., p. 256.
14. David Dilks, *Curzon in India, Vol. 1: Achievement and Vol. 2: Frustration*, (London: Rupert Hart Davis, 1969).
15. Peter King, *The Viceroy's Fall: How Kitchener Destroyed Curzon*, (London: Sidgwick and Jackson, 1986), pp. 98–102.
16. Winston S. Churchill, *Great Contemporaries*, (London: Leo Cooper, 1990 [1932]), pp. 173–84.

17. Richard J. Evans, *In Defence of History*, (London: Granta Books, 1997), p. 3.

18. Nigel Nicolson, *Mary Curzon*, p. 195.

19. D.H. Wrong, *Power*, (Oxford: Basil Blackwell, 1991), p. 124.

20. Wrong, *Power,* p. 125.

21. S. Gopal, *British Policy in India*, p. 227.

22. Gilmour, *Curzon,* p. 136.

23. Dilks, *Frustration,* p. 180.

24. Michel Foucault, *Selected Interviews*, C. Godard (ed.) (Brighton: Harvester, 1980), p. 156.

25. See, for instance, Arnold P. Kaminsky, *The India Office, 1880-1910* (London: Mansell, 1986), p. 73.

26. Keith Dowding, *Power*, (Buckingham: Open University Press, 1996), p. 4.

27. Dowding, *Rational Choice and Political Power*, (Aldershot: Edward Elgar, 1991), pp. 56–7.

28. 'Hamilton to Curzon', 14 August 1903, Curzon Papers, Mss Eur F111/162.

29. 'Ampthill to Curzon', 04 April 1902, Curzon Papers, Mss Eur F111/205.

30. P. Morriss, *Power: A Philosophical Analysis*, (Manchester: Manchester University Press, 2002 [1987]), p. 39.

31. Dowding, *Rational Choice and Political Power*, p. 157.

32. John R.P. French and Richard Synder, 'Leadership and Interpersonal Power', in *Studies in Social Power*, Dorwin Cartwright (ed.), (Ann Arbor: University of Michigan, 1959), 141.

33. Ibid., p. 139.

34. For example, see, Richard W. Davis, 'We Are All Americans Now!' Anglo-American Marriages in the Later Nineteenth Century. Proceedings of the American Philosophical Society, 135:2 (1991), p. 142.

35. Nigel Nicolson, *Mary Curzon*, pp. 72, 107.

36. John Kenneth Galbraith, *Anatomy of Power*, (London: Hamish Hamilton, 1984), pp. 47–9.

37. 'Mackworth Young to Mary', 14 October 1901, Curzon Papers, Mss Eur F111/230.

38. Richard Farndon (ed.), 'Introduction: A Sense of Relevance', in *Power and Knowledge: Anthropological and Sociological Approaches*, (Edinburgh: Scottish Academic Press, 1985), p. 6.

39. Max Weber, *On Charisma and Institution Building*, S.N. Eisenstadt (ed.), (Chicago: University of Chicago Press, 1968), 46.

40. R.F. Khan, 'A Note on the Concept of Authority', in *Leadership and Authority: A Symposium*, Gehan Wijeyewardene (ed.), (Singapore: University of Malaya Press, 1968), p. 7.

41. Edward VII to Brodrick, 20 February 1902, in Simon Heffer, *Power and Place: The Political Consequences of King Edward VII*, (London: Phoenix, 1999), p. 119.

42. 'Denzil Ibbetson to Curzon', 26 April 1904, Curzon Papers, Mss Eur F111/209.

43. Galbraith, *Anatomy of Power,* pp. 57–8.
44. Sir Walter Lawrence, *The India We Served,* (London: Cassell and Co., 1928), p. 252.
45. For a true-to-form analysis, see Bernard S. Cohn, *Colonialism and its Forms of Knowledge: The British in India*, (Princeton/Chichester: Princeton University Press, 1996), *passim* and Francis, *Governors and Settlers*, pp. 30–70.
46. J.C. Harsanyi, 'Measurement of Social Power, Opportunity Costs and the Theory of Two-Person Bargaining Games', in *Official Power: A Reader*, R. Bell et al. (eds.), (London: Collier-Macmillan, 1969), pp. 229–30.
47. Stewart Clegg, *Power, Rule and Domination*, (London: Routledge & Kegan Paul, 1975), p. 49.
48. Weber, *On Charisma*, p. 46.
49. Richard Sennett, *Authority*, (New York: Alfred A. Knopf, 1980), p. 46.
50. Manfred Kochen and Karl W. Deutsch, *Decentralization: Towards a Rational Theory*, (Cambridge, Mass./Konigstein: Gunn & Hain/Verlag Anton Hain, 1980), p. 16.
51. C. Friedrich, *Constitutional Government and Democracy*, (New York: W.W. Norton, 1941), Ch. 2, p. 57.

2

The India Office

An insider on the Council of India:

Godley: His only fault is that the Treasury Prig creeps up in him.

Alfred Lyall: Love of exercising power, which makes him love to intervene in a controversy. . . . Flattery, works wonders with him.

Sir James Peile: Hopelessly conventional . . . his maxim is that the most crusted Civil Service view is the right one.

Sir Charles Crosthwaite: Very great energy and ability, but most hostile.

Sir Steuart Bayley: An old dear, but indolent . . . sees the unreasonableness of the routine view of India . . .

Sir Dennis Fitzpatrick: A walking embodiment of all that you have ever said about the Punjab Government . . . entangled by precedents of his own making.

Sir J. Mackay: A great authority on finance and very able. . . . Amused [at] the crack he perpetrated when he assured you the Finance Committee were ignorant of your personal interest in certain proposals.

Sir John Edge: Very wise and able.

Sir P. Hutchins: Most liberal minded of the lot after Bayley.

Sir J. Westland . . . is Sir J. Westland.[1]

— Sir Richmond Ritchie to Curzon,
23 August 1901

The India Office was the body that followed Curzon's progress in India with the greatest interest, and was also by far the greatest constraint on Curzon's freedom of action as Viceroy. The interest may be attributed to the fact of its being Curzon's ultimate superior, and its sheer size, consisting as it did of the Secretary of State, the Permanent

Under-Secretary, the Council of India and the fact that during Curzon's time it had evolved close links with the British Cabinet. 'The real friend of India,' Curzon announced, 'will aim at the co-ordination of these powers'[2]—the Secretary of State and the Cabinet, the India Council and the Viceroy and his Council. But the process of coordination was not always smooth. Prima facie this was because the many components of the India Office had to consider the implications of Curzon's reforms with respect to myriad areas of polity, and thus tended to assess the Viceroy's plans from angles other than the purely Indian.

As far as the governance of India was concerned, the India Office's authority was ultimate and overreaching; it had a fiat over polity decisions made by other parties sharing administrative power in the governance of India; it was the office which had the final say, and tied up all loose ends in Indian administration. Apart from the obvious focus on policy as it was built up from Viceregal Lodge, studies of British policy in India tend to place an emphasis on pan-Empire politics, or the Imperial ideology as shapers of polity, especially in the period under scrutiny, *viz.*, the late nineteenth century: 'the manner in which Indian governmental business was processed and evaluated by Whitehall has been by and large ignored.'[3] The labyrinthine structure of the Home Government brought about a conflation of personal and constitutional struggles for supremacy and this affected Viceregal ability to legislate freely. While studying the India Office's relationship with their proconsul it is necessary to separately assess the reasons behind the prickly Curzon—Secretary of State equation, and the views of the India Council in relation to Curzon's Indian policy, as these two components were often driven by very different interests. It is also necessary to combine the lateral and the chronological views of Curzon's relationship with the India Office, as the Viceroy ran into obstacles of officialdom not only over persons, but also over planning. 'London' or 'Whitehall' in the context of the governance of India and with regard to constitutional authority over the Viceroy of India, had two major components: the Home Government (or more properly the British Cabinet) and the India

Office and its internal divisions and departments. While the Home
Government of course had ultimate control, the India Office could not
be ignored as they were the channel through which Parliament kept itself
informed about Indian affairs. And further, as Copland has observed,
'the effectiveness of Whitehall as an arbiter of Indian policy largely
depended on the capacity of the Secretary of State, and on the experience
and local knowledge [of the] . . . Council of India.'[4] But the 'India
Office' was not a homogenous entity, its myriad constituent offices,
individuals and councils and committees all being possessed of a highly
individualistic character.

The triangular equations between Curzon, the successive Secretaries of
State (George Hamilton and William St. John Brodrick) and the long-
serving Permanent Under-Secretary of State for India, Sir Arthur Godley,
later Lord Kilbracken, best showcase how inter-personal relations and
interests affected Curzon's reform drive. Hamilton's tenure in office is
emblematic of how the Secretary of State could liaise between Curzon,
the Permanent Under-Secretary and the British Cabinet, interposing his
vouchsafing of the Viceroy's prowess to maintain a universally amenable
balance of power between these often competing blocks of government.
Conterminously, St. John Brodrick's time in office showcases Curzon's
relations with his constitutional superiors against the backdrop of an
increasingly tempestuous Viceregal equation with the then British
Cabinet. The balance of power within the India Office after 1903 also
evidences how underlings might wield behind-the-scenes influence and
thus tailor the public image of individuals so as not to bring about
any rapprochement between antagonistic parties. A Viceroy, then, had
not only to contend with his Secretary of State's possibly contrarian
opinions on polity; he had also to contend with the machinations
that accompanied the internal workings of the India Office and the
Secretary of State's need to accommodate these. The Viceroy's position
in this set-up was anomalous. There existed two distinct streams of the
Government of India, the administrative and the political, and both
streams were concentrated in his persona. Additionally, the Viceroy also

had to handle the role of being the representative of a constitutional monarch. As Governor General he ruled India on behalf of the Crown. But, as Curzon himself pointed out, 'the latter title has no statutory sanction, and is the result merely of usage and convention.'[5] In practical terms, ruling India on behalf of the sovereign meant doing so on behalf of HM's Government of Great Britain. But the Viceroy was not directly responsible to the British Cabinet; he was instead answerable to the person of the Secretary of State for India, who liaised between the Viceroy and the Cabinet. The Secretary of State may have been the ultimate arbiter on India policy, and possessed all the powers conducive to autocratic rule, but the existence of the India Council checked this untrammelled exercise of authority, and supplied him with a 'constitutional obligation to conduct Indian business as a corporate entity—the Secretary of State in Council.'[6] The India Council, while composed of retired ICS men, may be considered an interest group analogous and subordinated to the India Office, partly because they were headed by the Secretary of State, and partly because many of them had no desire to see systems which they estimated had worked perfectly well in their day overturned by a new and zealous Viceroy, and thus tended to side with the Home Government in curbing some of Curzon's more enthusiastic schemes. The Secretary of State was also constrained in his responses to a Viceroy's concerns after taking into account how his response would be perceived by *his* superiors, the British Cabinet; as Clinton Dawkins opined about George Hamilton, 'Lord George [Hamilton] and Godley are properly enthusiastic about your great work in India, and are determined to back you up, though in the case of Lord George the determination is qualified by an apprehensive eye on Parliament and the PM.'[7] For the Secretary of State, as an appointee of the Prime Minister, did not operate either by himself or in a political vacuum; he was part of the body politic of the British Parliament. This analogy may be extended to the India Office in its entirety; even as it was an overseeing body, it was not a sovereign entity, and was itself answerable to Parliament. Under the circumstances, its interests in the Viceregal office may be said to primarily have been how Curzon's decision might affect the foreign relations and economic situation of the Empire as a whole. And, very obviously, what they perceived to be their interests altered and shifted with the individuals who occupied office. Officially, however, they were in denial about this; the Government was idealised as functioning independently of the entities who ran it; Godley urged Ampthill to recognise that the government 'is immortal, and incapable of "suspended animation," and that we cannot *officially* recognise the absence of any individual as a sufficient reason for postponing business or modifying decisions.'[8]

The dichotomies thus engendered were all the more pronounced in a Viceroy like Curzon, who was part of the parliamentary elite but chose not to conventionally participate in it by going off to the colonies. It is unsurprising that he appeared, alternatively, as a 'divinity addressing black beetles', and a breaker of ranks among those who put the Empire, as opposed to India, first. The situation was exacerbated by the fact that the India Office did not appoint the Viceroy; he was elected through informal consensus among the Cabinet and the governing elite. In Curzon's case, the then Secretary of State George Hamilton was only informed of his appointment when it had become a *fait accompli*. This rather convoluted practice of a (usually) member of the aristocracy appointed by a popularly elected British government administering a colony on behalf of the sovereign may have worked very well for the white dominions, where it gave the incumbent Governor General a degree of autonomy from Whitehall, which presumably allowed him to listen more to that Dominion's local government. It might also have worked excellently in places like Egypt, Sudan, and much of Africa, where proconsuls in relatively recently acquired colonies tended to be soldiers as opposed to statesmen. But in late Victorian India, the principle of consulting tiers of local government did not really apply; the Viceroy was expected either to implement or initiate polity. And putting a parliamentarian, one moreover fluent in constitutionalisms, into the proconsul's seat, and that too someone who had specialised in his charge, set the stage for a clash of authority between Whitehall and Simla.

Curzon's first finance member Clinton Dawkins once wrote him a succinct and fascinating account about how the various elements in power judged him as Viceroy, basing their judgements not only on their analysis of his performance, but also on how their co-judges viewed him; the already unwieldy tiers of authority built around the Viceroy gained a further volatility given the intrusion of interpersonal equations.[9] For the first four years of his Viceroyalty, the Secretary of State was George Francis Hamilton, who brought to the office over three years' experience by the time Curzon came to the Viceroyalty, but it was more than that: Hamilton was interested in the India Office for its own sake, for his successor St. John Brodrick, whom Curzon was to accuse of always trying to 'assert an untimely and inconsiderate exercise of superior power,'[10] it was a colourless political appointment like any other, and he could not share Curzon's passionate devotion to Indian affairs, over and above, of course, the frictional intrusion of their long running personal relationship. In the earlier half of Curzon's term, there was no obvious power bloc in London; Hamilton liaised between Curzon, the Permanent Under-Secretary of State, and the British Cabinet and India Council. Maintaining this delicate balance of power was crucial to Curzon's early successes. Post-1903, Curzon's relations with Whitehall became increasingly acrimonious as he encountered ever more opposition as his superiors asserted themselves and claimed primacy for their ideas about the governance of India.

While constitutionally the divisions and hierarchies, the spheres and levels of power were clearly demarcated, the conflicts as to who would have the final say arose largely as the result of a divide between 'man on the spot expertise', a concept normally championed by constitutional underlings, versus the desire to appropriate constitutionally sanctioned rights to superiority. The India Office's view of their status regarding the administration of India vis-à-vis the Viceroy was as follows: the Secretary of State for India, the head of the India Office, reported to the Cabinet, who were answerable to Parliament, which of course formulated policy after due regard for public opinion. Within the India Office, the

Secretary of State might communicate the Cabinet's views to the Viceroy direct, or he might do so after consultation with the Council of India, who could, of course, themselves recommend whether a Viceroy's ideas were worth assenting to. In such a linear hierarchy of power, it was extremely difficult for a Viceroy to be an originator of policy, much less to see it carried through the legislative process.

For itself, the India Office thus not only assumed its constitutional rights over the Viceroy, ultimately deriving its legitimacy from 'the people' but also endorsed several entities within its structure to exercise that right at different levels. At least three bodies—the India Office (as represented in the person of Godley), the Secretary of State, and the India Council—could directly override the Viceroy independently of each other. Curzon's view, understandably, was rather different.

CONTEXT OF THE LONDON–SIMLA RELATIONSHIP

Thus, as the Viceroyalty progressed, the core issue between Curzon and the London team actually became the balance of power and who would or could exercise more influence over Indian polity, and not, as in Hamilton's time, how declamations of authority could best be worked around to ensure the smooth functioning of government. Because of all the complex relationships of official and personal commingling, the issues discussed between the India Office and Simla, as between Simla and the provinces (though rather less so), centred around power and money, as opposed to legislation, especially of the welfare variety. As to Curzon's reforms, they became issues utilised in the tug of war. The debate over centralization, for instance, should merely have been a means to decide how best India should be governed, and not made an end in itself. This tended to overshadow actual questions of polity, as happened with the Kitchener affair. It is notable that after 1903, with the formation in London of a distinct power bloc consisting of the Secretary of State, the Permanent Under-Secretary—a post occupied by Sir Arthur Godley since 1883—and the Cabinet, with very specific aims and interests, very divergent from those of Curzon's simplistic and uni-dimensional ideals about improving the administration in India, Curzon's relations with Whitehall became increasingly acrimonious, and ended in his ouster. In part, however, it was also a matter of circumstance; by the time George Hamilton resigned over the issue of free trade, and Brodrick succeeded to the office the major reform pending (in the sphere of what would most concern Home, because it might infringe on the Empire as a whole) was that of the army. Brodrick *had* an interest in blocking Curzon's ideas because he was convinced Kitchener was right, and also wished to assert himself as a military tactician. Chief among the issues fought over was Centralization, in fact, it and the Kitchener affair, along with Curzon's relations with the India Council, were what concerned the Secretary and Permanent Under-Secretary to the exclusion of almost all else, certainly to the nitty-gritty of Curzon's reforms. The India Council's concerns were rather different, but they will be explored below.

The Constitutional Setting—Relationship with Curzon as Viceroy

Historians have contended that Curzon's Viceroyalty was 'perhaps the last time British policy in Asia was initiated not from Whitehall but from Calcutta,'[11] but this is debatable. It is probable that India's foreign policy was initiated (against opposition from London) from Calcutta, but the domestic policy, especially the financial side, came increasingly under the purview of Whitehall. The rationale for this strict scrutiny was that the Viceroy was too intent on a programme of centralization, or 'over centralization' as it was dubbed by its detractors. The India Office opposed centralization because it would, according to them, concentrate too much power in the hands of the Viceroy, and not because of any impact it may have had on the efficiency of administration in India. The India Office was against it, the India Council was against it[12] quite as much as the Governors of Bombay and Madras were against it, perhaps more so, and some of the provincial governors took care to enlist the India Office's support in their crusade against centralization.[13]

A great many personages were against it given that the initiative stemmed from someone generally acknowledged as not being a good team player, and thus it becomes imperative to examine how power struggles between London and Simla expressed themselves in debates over centralization.

Centralization crops up early in the Curzon–Godley correspondence, in just Godley's fourth letter to the Viceregal team of Curzon and Lawrence. But he chose to put it in a roundabout way, weaving it in with concerns over Bombay's lack of communication to London and Simla; 'No one, except myself, can be much less anxious than Lord Elgin was that the Supreme Government should grab the powers of the local governments, and, if he complained, we may be pretty sure that matters had gone too far;'[14] in the provincial autonomy direction, that is. Of course, emphasising the India Office's status as the ultimate law-maker on Indian affairs, and making it the point of reference for all government bodies in India was the apex of 'centralization', but this point seems to have been overlooked by Godley, Brodrick and the anti-centralization members on the India Council.

The view in London seems to have been that by taking a contrary line to the government policy on 'centralization', Curzon was insufficiently subordinate and not respectful of the constitutionalisms as to his ultimately underling position with regard to the Secretary of State. *Au contraire*, it may be that he recognised early on how a Viceroy could be thwarted by the Secretary of State and the India Council, and the subsequent need to co-opt them into any decision-making process early on. As he saw it, these two entities were what bounded a Viceroy's otherwise unfettered power: 'the head of the Government of India has more power than any other British subject.[15] He has the check of the Secretary of State and India Council, of course, but if he is a wise man (and Curzon very patently did not perceive himself as being other than wise!), he works with, and not in independence of them. There is no other official, or quasi-official check. . . .'[16]

This, of course, was not quite the view taken by the India Office. They in turn viewed themselves as being trust holders for the British Cabinet, Parliament, and ultimately the British people, and answerable to them as regards Indian affairs, a point Godley never failed to reiterate over and over again to Curzon. In addition to which Godley thought the Government of India too was not supportive of 'us' i.e., him and the British Government: 'Our policy would be greatly enhanced if you in India, instead of looking with jealousy upon the schemes which are submitted and taking up . . . an obstructive position, were to facilitate and encourage the work. . . .'[17] It may be observed that the India Office, by this attitude, ultimately wished to actively emphasise the British Government's role as the ultimate originator and arbiter about Indian legislation.

This goal was imperative for both Balfour and Brodrick. The base issue was power. Towards the end of Curzon's first term, he was seen as a hero not only in England, but also in India, by the Indians. His political rivals in England therefore bruited about 'that I have become too powerful, that I do not fall in readily enough with the views of the Cabinet, who would prefer a more docile Viceroy and a more slavish Council (i.e., a more slavish Viceroy's Council, though at this time London's chief complaint was the Viceroy's Council was much too complaisant with the Viceroy's wishes, and therefore slavish to the wrong authority), that I am regarded with jealousy and dislike by an India Council in England, who are conscious of a derogation from their former authority, and that I am even a source of disquietude to a Secretary of State who is anxious to assert his own individuality.'[18] They could not afford to be personally upstaged by Curzon, lest it affect their political fortunes. This interesting viewpoint throws up the contention that it was not merely a case of personal equations misfiring, but rather clashing lusts for power. Possibly both Balfour and Brodrick viewed Curzon's Viceroyalty as merely a prelude to the English premiership, and suspected that a glowing reputation in India might feed his success at Home. Hamilton was not possessed of the same overarching political ambition, and was thus untroubled by the fact that a successful Viceregal tenure would enhance Curzon's political stature at Home. The irony was that Curzon and Mary themselves seemed to think that a successful proconsul risked being stereotyped as a colonial administrator, and would thus not be taken seriously were he to make a bid for high office at Home. In any case, Curzon's actions as Viceroy were not carried out with one eye upon Downing Street.

Furthermore, as the people responsible for the ultimate direction of Indian affairs in Parliament, Balfour and his office were probably justified in fearing that ultimate control of India was being wrenched away from them, even though it was their prerogative; in theory this should not have mattered, given that Curzon was from the same political affiliation as the ruling government. It was here where Curzon's championing of the Indian cause began to play a part. Neither Balfour nor Brodrick was an expert in Indian affairs, and both had their reasons for wanting a smooth political ride. Balfour was leading a shaky government, and Brodrick was looking for a chance to redeem himself after an error-prone stint at the War Office. Indian affairs did not enthral the public, and moreover, Curzon's enthusiastic drives for justice and fairness only suggested that the government had hitherto been letting things slide in India. Moreover, it was the Army that Curzon's very public justice campaigns went after (since inter-departmental memos as to improving the extant work culture stayed internal and did not leak out to the press in England), and this had the ability (as demonstrated at the Durbar) to strike a chord with a public not overly sympathetic to Indian rights.

But, as pointed out above, neither of them had Indian backgrounds, or long experience in running Indian affairs and they needed a front man who could negotiate through the labyrinthine links between Indian administrators, returned and former, to rein in Curzon. And they, especially St. John, had always been conscious of their having plodded their way into government as opposed to Curzon's diametric rise. Brodrick was still acutely aware of his 'intellectual inferiority', and tried to validate himself on that count, thus seeking to justify to himself and to Curzon, the circumstances by which he had become Curzon's constitutional superior. It was widely known that he did not have any specific interest in India, unlike his predecessor, but he claimed that his previous stint at the War Office was more than germane, especially under the contemporary circumstances. 'You think me wholly lacking in Indian experience,' he wrote to Curzon at the height of the Kitchener affair, 'whereas having spent nearly fifteen years dealing directly with soldiers, I . . . have . . . a greater knowledge of their idiosyncrasies . . . than any Civilian.'[19] Curzon, it was well known, had nothing but contempt for the military, and the Indian army at that point of time in particular, for a man who had dedicated a work on the frontier to the army, Curzon had managed to make himself extremely unpopular with it much before Kitchener ever set foot in India.

ATTITUDES OF ARTHUR GODLEY

What was indubitably Balfour's and Brodrick's to command, however, was Godley, often described as the power behind the thrones of successive Secretaries of State, and the hand who controlled how the Viceroys would be judged in England. Godley was a major obstacle in Curzon's winning over the India Office, not only because he exercised an out-of-proportion influence within it, but also because he used his considerable clout to swing opinion around. He seems to have craved power—not power in the absolute, but influence over those who occupied the highest posts. At the same time he does not seem to have wished to jeopardize his political careers by criticising those he saw to be in comparative favour with his own superiors. But he was reluctant to expose himself to positions of unfamiliar responsibility; in 1903 Curzon asked him to take up the post of Finance Member of the Council of India, but Godley refused, noting however that, 'the fun [of the offer] consist[ed] in the fact that the appointment was not in the Viceroy's gift, but in that of the Secretary of State.'[20] This pinpoints just how much he valued his behind-the-scenes post, and regarded others as mere pretenders when it came to the exercise of authority and the patronising of high office. Certainly the division of Indian responsibilities and the place of the Viceroy in the hierarchy of Indian government began to be more and more scrutinised by Godley only in the post-Hamilton era:

> The relations between the Secretary of State and the Viceroy are peculiar, and, if they are to be maintained on an agreeable footing, it is very desirable that both of those high officials should be endowed with an adequate amount of tact and of what Matthew Arnold called 'sweet reasonableness'. For in India the Viceroy is a sublime autocrat, . . . and yet he is under the thumb of the Secretary of State, who has absolute power over him. . . .[21]

The implication, of course, being that the Secretary of State was more powerful than the most powerful person in the Indian Empire: Godley's comment betrays a sense of gloating at his boss' having power over the person who had power over 300 million people; hence, power over 300 million plus one souls. Not to speak of the administrative apparatus of British India (which at that point did not include many of the 300 million Indian souls, but was almost exclusively British) that existed to carry out the orders of the Viceroy.

In addition, Godley seems to have regarded Curzon much as one might regard an over-enthusiastic novice. Over and over again he reiterated that because the Secretary of State, the Prime Minister and the Cabinet had 'absolute and unshared responsibility' for every one of Curzon's acts, there must be a corresponding right of control, absolute and unshared, over Curzon's actions by these personages.[22] While Godley is often portrayed—with some justification—as the villain behind the scenes who was responsible for leaving Curzon politically isolated over the Kitchener affair by most Viceregal biographers, it would seem that, towards the close of the Conservative government's time in office, he, and his known anti-Curzon views, were used by Balfour and Brodrick to voice hard truths to the Viceroy, matters which would have been unpleasant for them to communicate.[23] It may of course be that Godley may have nursed similar views all along, and only repressed them when serving under George Hamilton, a staunch supporter of Curzon. Certainly he was effusive in his praise of Brodrick, something he did not accord to Hamilton; 'With Brodrick my own relations were most agreeable throughout the two years that he spent with us. . . . I found him . . . remarkably easy and pleasant to work with.'[24] Certainly, towards the spring of 1905, when Curzon's relations with Balfour and Brodrick were collapsing, Godley became ever more hectoring and openly disapproving of the Viceroy: 'I also . . . dissociate myself from any censure which you might be inclined to pass upon the way in which Members of Council have used their powers . . . as to the general iniquity of their conduct I am quite sure that we should not agree.'[25] Or it may just have been self-preservation; either way, Godley shows up as an agile political chameleon. He even tried to take credit for the 'partition' of Bengal, writing to Curzon that, 'This is a tremendously big thing that you have achieved, and I am only sorry that you will not be there yourself to carry the scheme into actual effect and practical working.[26] As you know I have myself from the first believed in your scheme, and felt sure that it would be carried, but without the vigorous help of the Secretary of State [blatant toadying to Brodrick] it might easily have been longer.'[27] It was not that Curzon was unaware of Godley's growing, and increasingly active hostility.

As relations between himself and the Cabinet deteriorated, and Godley fanned the flames, the Viceroy tried to point out how Godley himself had not always been uncritical of the Home establishment, writing to him that 'a good deal of my evidence as to their attitude has been supplied (at any rate in earlier times) by yourself.'[28] Godley had in fact sympathised at times with Curzon's struggles with the India Council, agreeing that that body needed an overhaul; but he had also sympathised with the Council over Curzon, and never tried to gloss over possible avenues for a breach between Curzon and his Secretaries of State. Godley's idea of ministering political support seems to have been expressed in deprecating those he felt would be regarded as threats or obstacles by his correspondents.

Brodrick's alleged mental stolidity may have played a greater part in determining the course of Curzon's Viceroyalty than merely setting him up to feel resentful towards his school friend; it may have prevented him from introspecting and contextually weighing Godley's opinions. It is possible he was sucked into Godley's view of Curzon as the reckless young man in a hurry because of the respect he accorded Godley on account of his long Indian experience. Godley was acutely aware that Curzon, though a part of the ruling establishment, was not regarded unambiguously by them at all and would thus never back the Viceroy, but always the India Council, because they at least were confirmed experts, and anyway not inclined to ruffle the feathers of the Government, as they were not rivals for current or future political pre-eminence. He said this to Curzon. 'I told [Curzon] . . . that I was "not much surprised" (I certainly was not) at his being vexed by the occasional obstacles . . . placed in his way [by the Council] . . . my expressions of sympathy were . . . preliminary to remarks intended to bring this truth home to him . . . he must not expect to get his way in everything. But he has a gift for reading . . . the meaning that he wants to find.'[29]

Being the recipient of these confidences, Hamilton of necessity had to play a balancing act, acting as an intermediary between Godley, the Council and the Viceroy, of whom he was genuinely fond. He seems to have succeeded admirably; it was after his departure as Secretary of State that relations between Curzon and Whitehall went steadily downhill: 'Since you left the India Office, I have met with little sympathy or support, and this has been the more galling when it has rested upon an ignorance of Indian Government and Indian conditions that is truly startling.'[30]

But it was not just Hamilton's comparatively superior knowledge of Indian affairs that contributed to Curzon's uncomplicated relationship with Hamilton—and the harmonious Viceroy—Secretary of State equation this established; this was in large part due to Hamilton deferring to Curzon's superior knowledge. According to S. Gopal, it did not pave the way for a similar camaraderie with A.J. Balfour and

St. John Brodrick, both of whom were 'not indifferent to the exercise of power.'[31] But Hamilton had been no pushover either when it came to defending the interests of 'Home'. The year 1902 in fact saw one of the few instances where Hamilton crossed Curzon with a degree of success, and it very nearly ended in Curzon's resignation. The issue was Curzon's proposed remission of the Salt Tax at the Coronation Durbar; while not strictly a piece of reform, it was one of Curzon's most cherished—and bitterly fought for—projects. For Curzon, it was perfectly in keeping with what he said was Oriental tradition, and a way of binding together the King and the people of the country, and on the strength of this reasoning he dispatched a sanguinary epistle outlining his plans to London. The horrified Hamilton at once shot it down, citing issues of precedent and protocol. Nevertheless, he felt obliged to furnish an explanation to the Viceroy stating he had not done so merely on the strength of his office—he had never tried to claim primacy for *ex-officio* authority over Curzon's specialist knowledge:

> I felt bound to consult the best authorities I could in the matter before I gave you any further answer. I showed your letter to Sir Arthur Godley; he is emphatic that your proposal is one which could not be assented to. I took the opinion of the Finance Committee: they all held the same view. I consulted the Chancellor of the Exchequer: he expressed himself equally strongly. I spoke to the Prime Minister . . . he was clearly of opinion that the objections, both financial and constitutional, to the course you suggested were almost insuperable . . . nothing would induce the Council here to assent to any such proposal; and, when you consider that they by Parliament are specially entrusted with the control of Indian finance . . . is it reasonable to suppose that they could properly give up the functions they are thus specially appointed to discharge, without a full and complete examination of what the financial resources and the expenditure requirements of the Indian Government are likely to be for the next few years?[32]

This did nothing to convince Curzon; he was not in the least impressed, he said, with the point about the precedent: 'Each Durbar is a law to itself, and both creates and extinguishes its own precedent.'[33] As to expert opinion, he dismissed talk of it being disinterested; upon hearing that the Council of India was unanimously against the proposal, without, it was stressed, being prompted to take such a line by the Secretary of State, he shot back that, 'Of course the India Council may be inspired exclusively by motives of financial orthodoxy or constitutional Puritanism . . . [but] the question of the Coronation guests in England caused, as you know, a great tension, and . . . it was in their power to take it out of me over the Delhi Durbar.'[34]

The final compromise—an announcement at the Durbar promising future concessions—only served to prove just how far Curzon was willing to accommodate contrarian opinions so as to continue in office and see out the implementation of the rest of his programme, and vice versa. A Viceroy with strong convictions was probably deemed to be a price worth paying to ensure good administration. This would not be the case three years later.

THE SECRETARIES OF STATE: HAMILTON, BRODRICK

For the present, however, there were deeper reasons than a prickly Viceregal pride that contributed to Curzon's progressively deteriorating clout with London; while both Hamilton and Brodrick were Conservative Secretaries of State, appointed by a Conservative Government, and liaising with a Conservative Viceroy, their periods in office were characterised by two very different political climes at Home. Hamilton had been Secretary of State for three years when Curzon became Viceroy, and thus did not run the risk of being called a rubber stamp Secretary of State even if he unhesitatingly endorsed every decision of Curzon's. Appointed by Salisbury, he was dealing with an old favourite ideological counterpart of the old Prime Minister, in what was the Conservative high noon. Brodrick came to office when the government, headed by Salisbury's nephew, and his and Curzon's long-time friend Balfour, was increasingly shaky, and he was sandwiched between two old school friends who had risen to eminence. Hence, it was not just due to personality clashes and ego issues that the Curzon–Brodrick relationship was much less smoother than the Curzon–Hamilton one.

The other major difference between the Secretary-ships of Hamilton and Brodrick, and perhaps a key to why they turned out so differently, may lie in the long association between Curzon and Brodrick. Hamilton approached the new Viceroy, whose enthusiastic forward policies contrasted sharply with his own advocacy of moderation,[35] with a degree of trepidation, and thus probably trod softly. It is possible that both Curzon and Brodrick, when in office, did not feel the need to infuse much 'officialdom' into their relationships; their frequent allusions to their schoolboy bonds hint that they may have relied too much on those bonds to forge an easy official relationship, envisaging it as an extension of their youth; and Curzon was probably also lulled by the confiding and confidential relationship he had had with Hamilton, and assumed a process of transference would see it continue with Hamilton's successor. But as Kenneth Rose notes, 'informal diplomacy, conducted rather in a code of common understanding than in the precise language of a state paper, is un-fitted for the determination of high policy.'[36] Further, when people known to each other clash in official capacities over questions of polity, 'a sense of betrayal poisons official relationships; whereas the chance acquaintances of a more democratic society can debate their differences on an austerely intellectual plane.'[37] The Curzon–Brodrick equation was weighted down with misguided expectations from both men even as it was formed.

And finally, the Curzon–Brodrick equation included a third party—their old fellow-Soul and then Prime Minister, Arthur James Balfour. Balfour was inextricably linked with Curzon's rocky relationship with St. John Brodrick. Balfour's biographers uniformly (in a holding pattern the diametric opposite of their 'others', the Curzon biographies) lay the blame on Curzon for the abrupt termination of the Curzon Viceroyalty and the strained relations with Balfour and Brodrick that followed. But they do bring into significance that Balfour, unlike Brodrick, had to consider the overall Government side of the picture. But ultimately, of all Curzon's political superiors who turned into his opponents over the Kitchener affair, Balfour was the one who maintained his regard for

Curzon's abilities throughout, also showing himself to be in some sympathy with the Viceroy's frustrations. For one, he did not take kindly to the India Council, stating that he did 'not believe in the elaborate system of check and counterchecks'[38] that the existence of the India Council inevitably engendered, and claimed to fully endorse the Viceroy's sense of being thwarted when plans long-thought-out by the Government of India were quashed promptly by the Council. But, ultimately, Balfour had no say in the matter because the India Council and Indian affairs generally were the parliamentary provenance of St. John Brodrick. And as Prime Minister, while he pondered on the possible fallout of Curzon's diplomatic missions, Balfour also had to contend with dissension within the India Office over Curzon's domestic policy. Freed from the moderating influences of George Hamilton, and guided by an increasingly sycophantic (towards St. John Brodrick) Arthur Godley, the India Council lost no opportunity to record its dissatisfaction with the Viceroy's centralization programmes and his alleged overriding of the ICS.

Certainly very different impetuses prompted Balfour and Brodrick's very different reactions towards Curzon. Many biographers have attributed Brodrick's non-support of Curzon to a secret jealousy at an old friend's greater success, but this motive cannot be supplied in the case of Balfour. It was Curzon's aggressive foreign policy that most seemed to irk Balfour, having inherited something of his uncle's latter-day caution and holding together a precarious Government. Balfour definitely did not share all of Curzon's enthusiasm for strengthening the imperial ideal, as his chief concern was holding on to power at Home, without risking it through gambles abroad. Dawkins' observation on how Balfour differed from Salisbury over Indian polity has already been reproduced above.[39] Dawkins' identification of Curzon's second bug bear was not to prove crucial to wrecking his Viceroyalty; Salisbury might or might not think Curzon was going too fast down the path of reform, and over centralizing,[40] but Dawkins' informant [of Salisbury's views] certainly would. However much St. John Brodrick passed on the gist of his conversations with his friend Balfour's uncle to Dawkins, his own views would be remarkably similar as Secretary of State. It is, of course, highly possible that both Balfour and Brodrick were persuaded as to the brinkmanship of Curzon's Indian foreign policy by Balfour's uncle and political mentor, the Marques of Salisbury—Balfour was always quoting Salisbury's comments about Curzon's advocacy of an aggressive Russian policy, as though his uncle's comments legitimised his own views about the Viceroy.

Balfour appeared to feel that an Indian Viceroy should be the instrument who carried out Whitehall's foreign policy instructions pertinent to the region. Curzon, if he had had his own way, would have pursued any independent line he thought was best for India's interests, and would have 'raised India to the position of an independent and not always friendly power.'[41] It was this 'insubordination' that Balfour and the governmental establishment raged against 'the Government condoned Curzon's shortcomings respecting Tibet and Afghanistan by sending him back to India, and on the other points by declining to accept his resignation (in June) . . . [even when] they and he disagreed on the question of the Military Member of the Council. . . .'[42] It would appear that the government expected Curzon to be grateful for having been given a rein freer than that had been given to most other Viceroys, but on the contrary, according to Balfour, 'no such public exhibition of disloyalty to the Home Government has ever yet been made by an Indian Viceroy.'[43]

A great deal of the debate between Curzon and the India Office, in fact, was characterised by protestations as to which of them had to do the most compromising and give in to the other's ideals, as well as which had the task with the greater gravity before them. Curzon may have thought that the Viceroy had his task cut out, a continent away from being able to justify his opinions in person to a Secretary of State always accessible to a hostile (to himself, according to Curzon's perception) India Council, but Brodrick was convinced it was the Secretary of State who carried the greater burden. 'I honestly think,' he lost no time in pointing out to Curzon, 'the position of Secretary of State is much more difficult in his relations with the Viceroy than those of the Viceroy with the Secretary of State . . . the Viceroy, under present conditions, monopolises all initiative. The Secretary of State consequently has to deal with subjects . . . brought to him by a very able body . . . with whom discussion is, for physical reasons, impossible. [He also] . . . has at his elbow . . . the Council [who] . . . are always less likely to agree with the Viceroy . . . he has also to deal with the Cabinet [who can] take a line perfectly independent of [the Viceroy's] opinion.'[44]

In turn, Curzon pointed out to Brodrick the desirability of listening to the (presumably) expert man on the spot: 'Hamilton once wrote to me that he would be most averse from overruling the unanimous opinion of the Viceroy and his Colleagues [sic] on any purely Indian matter, i.e., on any matter which did not present Imperial aspects, in which case of course the Home Government must be supreme.'[45] It is evidence of how, by 1905, it was high politics rather than Indian polity that was foremost in the minds of those governing India from London, that they assumed even Curzon was fighting the proposed military reforms out of a desire to retain personal control over the system; to reassure him, Balfour wrote to him that, 'one thing I am sure it [the new system] will not do; it will not diminish the authority which the Governor General has over matters of army as well as of Civilian administration.'[46]

It is therefore apparent that there was no unanimous consensus as to the importance to be accorded to Curzon's views and ideas about Indian administration among the highest echelons of power in Whitehall. This was starkly manifested after he resigned. Opinions were cleanly divided as to how he should be treated on his return. Brodrick (and Godley) did not want Curzon to get an honour (the peerage customarily bestowed on retiring Viceroys) because such an act might be read by the public as implying that the King's sympathies were with Curzon and not the British Government (for by this time they spoke of themselves as opposites).[47] Balfour, however, was strongly in favour of the move; he could 'not agree with those (if there be any such) who think that any differences he may so far have had with the Government, cancel his claims to their regard.'[48] But Brodrick's writing to Knollys, quoting excerpts from the press which vilified Curzon, was more than a pitched attempt to have him denied a peerage and so (according to Brodrick's line of thinking) embarrass the Government. Brodrick, deliberately or otherwise, did more than actively undermine a source of power that Curzon might have clung to on his return; without it, he was out of politics for the next six years, and more pertinently, not in a position to influence Indian affairs. The British Government at Home had made the point that, in the event of a clash, its views, and not the Government of India's, carried primacy when it came to Indian legislation.

So it may be said that the India Office was not interested in Curzon's reforms per se: they were interested in implementing current governmental policy in India, and if that clashed with Curzon's reforms, they were happy to ditch the reforms and George. For quite different reasons, a government which did not always support its man in India found an ally in the India Council.

THE INDIA COUNCIL: COMPOSITION, ATTITUDES

In contrast to the many theories that have grown up around the India Office's more visible *dramatis personae's* reluctance to endorse Curzon's Viceregal polity, it has not been felt necessary to investigate, beyond the obvious, the causes which compelled the India Council to object to many of the Viceroy's reforms; this was after all an entity traditionally portrayed as an identikit corpus of the retired heaven-born, nursing crabbed jealousies of an incumbent Governor General who had risen higher in India than they had ever done or could ever hope to.[49] In fact, the Councillors and the role they should be accorded in the shaping of policy were a major bone of contention between Curzon and Godley. According to Clinton Dawkins, the India Council was one of the two major forces from which Curzon would meet opposition for his reforms, even though Hamilton managed to neutralize or evade their [the India Council's] opposition most of the time. Newcomers were often astonished by the vitriol; Sir Hugh Barnes took his seat on the Council in May 1905 at the height of the Kitchener affair, straight away upon his return from Burma. The Council in spirit was probably supposed to act as a benevolent advisory body, helping run the administration of India smoothly, and Sir Hugh professed himself:

much astonished at the . . . hostility to . . . Your Excellency . . . assumed by several members of Council. Lee-Warner is of course always controversial and excitable, and his chief craze is that you are a terrible autocrat . . . that the members of the Viceroy's Council are non-entities . . . highly dangerous and unconstitutional [situation]. Fitzpatrick is the worst . . . always inputting motives, generally unworthy ones.

He went on to hope that his own presence would have some kind of salutary effect: 'that someone with recent knowledge stands up to . . . antiquated old members . . . will have its effect.'[50] Curzon had wanted him on the Council as a counterpoise to Sir William Lee-Warner, because 'his political knowledge will correct many of the vagaries of Lee-Warner, while he has considerable all-round experience, charming manners, and great tact.'[51] Further, a person who was just back from India could provide a very valuable continuum of policy, and assess events in a contemporary context, and make the transition from Viceroy to Viceroy easier.

This last was especially important because the Council was not just antagonistic to Curzon on its own behalf; its 'tendency to oppose [was] stimulated by hints and correspondence from . . . people in India . . . who dislike change and dislike the pain of new ideas;'[52]—the Lieutenant Governors and the ICS men Curzon managed to upset with his ideas for reform. The council, under the leadership of Alfred Lyall, of course looked upon these missives as proof that their policies and legacies were still going strong among those who might have served under them during the course of their Indian careers. This is not to suggest that the Council was homogeneous. Councillors held vastly differing opinions, and aired them with unequal degrees of conspicuousness and effect. The first Council of Curzon's Viceroyalty was headed by George Hamilton as Secretary of State, and otherwise consisted of Sir S. Bayley, Sir J. Peile, Sir C. Crosthwaite, Sir F. Le Merchant, Sir D. Fitzpatrick, Sir J. Mackay, Sir J. Edge and Sir P. Hutchins.[53] As Secretary of State Hamilton presided over the Council whenever it met; they met regularly at weekly intervals.

The individual views and stances of the individual Councillors, however, did not result in the formation of power blocs within the Council over the issue of military reform; the final explosive break-up of the Viceroyalty had nothing to do with the Council or the Councillors, and everything with the nature of the Curzon–Godley–Brodrick triangle. The reason for this, of course, is that the termination of Curzon's Viceroyalty owed much to high politics, and over appointments not within the sphere of the ICS and thus traditionally not within the purview of the India Council, who dealt with matters of civil administration only. Many Councillors were very vocal about it—in private correspondence. However, by the time 1905 rolled around, the Council of India was undergoing a major change in composition, most of the established members such as Lyall—he had served on the Council for fifteen years—Crosthwaite, Bayley, MacDonnell, Peile having retired, and Sir Hugh Barnes having only just assumed MacDonnell's place after having retired from the Lieutenant Governorship of Burma in mid-1905. It was probably at its weakest in terms of political clout than at any other point during Curzon's Viceroyalty. Thus, curiously, a Council whose alleged over-interference had been the major source of conflict between Curzon and Godley (and perhaps ultimately turned Godley away from Curzon) did not play any part in the summer of 1905. It is as though after being pinpointed as a 'deal breaker' up to 1903–04, the Council subsides quietly into the dust as the Kitchener affair gathers steam. The Minutes of the Council by their silence with regards to the Kitchener Affair become important. They provide an understanding of how the civilian-military conflict between the Viceroy and the Commander-in-Chief played out in London. The role of the Council

of India in the Kitchener–Curzon dispute has yet to be fully investigated;
why did they, arguably one of the major thwarters of the Viceroy's plans
for administrative reforms, apparently stay silent when confronted with
an issue of great political and administrative magnitude? The only
apparent notation about the controversy is a Minute regarding it as
closed, as of 25 July 1905—at which time it did appear that Curzon
and Kitchener had reached a working compromise. It is worth noting
here that the Minutes of the meeting which assembled immediately
following Curzon's resignation contain any references to the event; either
it was not discussed, or left off the record. The Secretary of State
Brodrick, who normally presided over the meeting by virtue of his office,
was conspicuously absent, the meeting being chaired by Sir P. Hutchins.

It is also possible that the Minutes of the Council do not reveal what
went on. As a Council the Councillors functioned as a block, and if one
or more dissented over a move, the Minutes note the dissension, but are
silent as to its cause. Thus, Sir H. Barnes' sympathy for Curzon over the
issue of Military administration is apparent only from his personal
correspondence; as a Member of Council his individual voice is not on
record. But the Council's relative silence over the Kitchener affair may
also be because the handling of the Kitchener Affair was supervised, and
largely conducted by, the Imperial Defence Committee instituted by
Balfour, and also because the Council as such was responsible for civilian
affairs of administration only. But the Council, because of its very role
as an advisory body, could have demanded a thorough discussion of the
Kitchener controversy as it dragged on, and did not. From their
comparative silence one can assume that the centre of power in this affair
was elsewhere.

While such an approach negates the fluid dynamics that operated within
the India Office, the situation was entirely in keeping with the class
dynamics through which the government of Great Britain was organised,
as well as the divide between civil and military administration.
Kitchener's appointment and the subsequent intriguing involved the War
Office, the British Cabinet and the Secretary of State and Godley merely

represented the India Office's views, because it was an Indian affair. The India Council, being civilians as well as socially and politically largely un-connected to the business of Home British government, might express their views insofar as they wanted to support or criticise the Viceroy's policy, but they had very little access to the sources of power and decision making at Whitehall. It is true, however, that some of the more prolific Councillors, such as Alfred Lyall and Lee-Warner, who would serve on the Council for a decade, made very public pronouncements on Curzon's policies and relations with the British Government, but the weight given to these was more due to their prominence in their Indian careers, than by virtue of the Councillor's offices they held. Thus, in the end, it emerged that any decisive turns and shifts in Indian polity would be dependent on political events to do with the Home Government, not with any of the constituent departments of the Government of India. The India Council was unobtrusively barred from the highest echelons of decision making in Indian polity.

The Council records are useful for understanding why a Secretary of State might have endorsed a move that he knew would not go down well in India, because he had taken the advice of the Council upon it and prioritised that over feedback from India. Given that the Council of India discussed all matters of administration that would have been similarly discussed by the Viceroy's Council in India, and even by the specific departments of provincial administrations in India, Curzon was probably justified in complaining about their tendency to pronounce, or reverse, judgements on issues without considering what other departments had had to say about those issues.[54] The Council discussed topics as wide ranging as the appointments and careers of the senior administrators of India, to the railway system in Bengal to the extant political situation on Tinnelvely District, which was, to say the least, disturbed. But it is difficult to understand how the India Council could effectively contribute constructively on matters as to which contractor was suitable for the Simla–Kalka rail at a 7000 kilometre remove.

The Council of India was also responsible for having communications from the Government of India conveyed to other departments which might need to be involved, mostly the Colonial Office. The mistreatment of Indians in South Africa was a case in point. It was one of the issues Curzon pursued most vigorously, and enquiries and directions as to the resolution of the matter were directed to the High Commissioner for South Africa via the Colonial Office via the Council of India/India Office. In this case the Council of India functioned as a liaising body for the Government of India and a link to departments in London which it would have been cumbersome to establish a separate line of communication with. This was undoubtedly useful but it did mean that the Council of India's status as a channel through which information flowed dictated that they could control that flow—something that the Government of India was perhaps right to resent. A body constituted merely for advisory purposes, supposed to hold no legislative power, and moreover, having no checks upon its deliberations, should not really have been placed in such a strong position vis-à-vis the Government of India, after all, the Council of India should not have been in the position of a rival claimant for access to power in London when it was intended to make the Government of India's task easier, not harder, which is what both Curzon and the people on the Council of India during his time seemed to wilfully set out to do.

While Curzon's coming to office, and the specific circumstances that surrounded it, did much to precipitate a crisis in smooth relations between the Viceroy and the India Council, these tensions had a base in past polity. The violent clashes between Curzon's predecessor Elgin, and the India Office would in themselves have provided enough impetus to increase the said office's guardedness towards its proconsuls. The lingering distaste of Elgin's perceived ineptness, coupled with the general alarm with which an enthusiastic Curzon's appointment was regarded, meant that the India Office was doubly wary by 1898. The uneasy relationship was exacerbated when Curzon made it very clear that he did not care for the India Council, the favoured advisors for the India

Office. Unfortunately for all concerned, none of Curzon's immediate predecessors had possessed specialist Indian knowledge, and the India Council had got used to having Viceroys who were suitably subservient to the specialists—the old India Hands. The India Council did not, of course, exercise much power in its own right. As regards Indian matters, it could be overruled by the Secretary of State. As to its members exercising power in the British governmental apparatus, this was not very likely as they mostly did not come from the ruling class, and were in any case, specialised Indian administrators as opposed to politicians. And as a matter of fact, because of the heightened pace of contemporary politics, matters of large administrative issues appear to have been debated upon in the British Cabinet as opposed to the India Council or even the India Office. But the Council could, of course, change the way a Viceroy was perceived by his contemporaries in Parliament, by backing (or not) his policies. By dropping hints to the Council via the Secretary of State, a Government could, therefore, dictate Indian polity if it was so minded to do. And when a Viceroy clashed with the Council, as Curzon did, whichever could prove themselves in the right to the Government would have the upper hand.

The relations between Curzon, Godley and Hamilton via the India Council are crucial to an understanding of the degree of success Curzon had in convincing people as to his plans, principally because it was the powers assigned to this Council that became the major bone of contention between Curzon and Whitehall. For the Secretary of State, and especially Godley, who had never been to India, the views of the India Council were a back-up that could be used to vindicate abstract government policies a Viceroy might bridle against, given that the India Council was supposed to consist of 'experts', moreover, of the type that would have had more direct experience of India than any Viceroy. For the incumbent Viceroy, on the contrary, the same reasons would make the Council a meddlesome irritant.

Thus, Curzon's relations with this body, while they do not seem to have greatly affected the administration of India—even though the Council had a veto vote in matters financial—did affect his relations with the Secretary and Permanent Under-Secretary of State for India, and this in turn affected how his reform schemes were received in London. Since the latter functionaries worked in close proximity to the India Council, and their own relations with it were often delicately balanced[55] Curzon's fulminations against the India Council affected them too. Further, the extent to which the Council's stamp was discernible on Indian polity reflected on the prowess and influence (with the Councillors) of the Secretary of State; Clinton Dawkins remarked to Curzon that one of the reasons for the Council, which was, after all, merely an advisory body intended to assist the Secretary of State in forming opinions, being so restive was that Hamilton could not exercise proper dominance over it, and when he did, often downplayed triumphs to keep the councillors from breaking out in rage.[56] But Hamilton's successor Brodrick seemed to have the Council behind him, and used the Councillors' public clout to swing opinion away from Curzon. But even Brodrick, generally disposed to back the Council over Curzon, admitted, however, that the Council of India, consisting as it did of 'several men with strong personality besides long Indian experience . . . were disposed to scrutinize with special care the changes and problems which Lord Curzon showered upon them. . . .'[57] It would seem that even those actually serving on the Council of India did not wholeheartedly approve of the nature of its functions; as Lyall, one of the more eminent councillors, whom Curzon had wanted for the Governorship of Bombay, put it: 'one can prevent some mischief, but do little good, on the Council.'[58] The Council, of course, did not have the power to initiate new legislation! A less 'political' reason behind Curzon's tempestuous relationship with the India Council may be the possibility that the Secretary and Permanent Under-Secretary of State relied thoroughly on advice from the Council, while the Viceroy felt his word should be the final one. Curzon's zeal for overhauling the administrative machinery may well have been viewed as too ambitious or unfounded by India veterans, and after all he did not have long experience of colonial governance to back up his claims, and this meant that the Council of

India, for reasons aforementioned, would be listened to. And, quite simply, it would also seem that Curzon was right about the India Council deriving its ideas from the ICS days of its constituent members; Lee-Warner, for instance, thought of the Bombay Presidency as an essentially politically unstable place (a view echoed by the then police chief A.H.L. Fraser in India), as opposed to Curzon, who actually seems to have inclined towards a rather positive assessment of the presidency and its people. And given that the Council was on the spot to influence the rest of the India Office, and the weightage of their collective expertise, any Secretary of State might be forgiven for taking their advice and not Curzon's when it came to the choosing.

Curzon himself very firmly saw the Council of India as being diametrically opposed to the Government of India, writing to Godley of 'your Council', and the obstructions it put up against 'our policy'. Curzon insinuated that the Council was being used as a front to wrest control of Indian affairs away from India: 'Under the new theory of Indian Government, internal affairs, popularly believed to be the main function of the Government of India, are also controlled by the majority of the India Council in London.'[59] Brodrick in turn felt this approach only served to further alienate the Council, and induce them to throw obstacles towards the realisation of the Viceroy's vision for India; 'because Curzon and the India Council did not get on, the Council started discussing things with greater freedom than they would otherwise have done.'[60] He expected the Council to be much more complaisant with the Government of India's demands once Ampthill had been installed as Acting Viceroy, but by then the Council was out of the equation insofar as the power stakes in the governance of India were concerned.

Despite such indicators, the India Council was not merely an anachronistic body, whose differences with Curzon were used as a clout-manipulator by the rest of the India Office and the British Cabinet. Hamilton was outspoken in his criticism of the Council's ways, and even Godley admitted in the wake of the 1882 famines that, 'there was a strong inclination on the part of the Council . . . to be parsimonious and to higgle [*sic*] over unimportant details in the making of contracts. . . .'[61] Chief among the Council's faults was the propensity—widely but probably not disapprovingly noted of—the Councillors to be somewhat reactionary and proprietary of Indian administration. Railway expansion was one of Curzon's pet—and most successful—schemes, but the India Council did not initially take too kindly to it; as a matter of fact the Councillors did not accede to his proposals, even though he had appointed a special Railway Commission. As Clinton Dawkins explained apologetically to the Viceroy, 'Lyall is the great obstacle to more generous treatment of Railway enterprise . . . he is the old Qui [*sic*] Hai . . . and reflects the old attitude against interlopers.'[62] One wonders who the interlopers were, presumably the forty-three year old Viceroy, who had by then held office for three-and-a-half years. Godley termed the all-round attitude to railway reform 'unsatisfactory', blaming the India Council for not backing it: 'members of the council . . . have the whip hand of the Secretary of State, and it is extremely difficult to get them to take a broad or statesmanlike view.'[63] According to Hamilton's private secretary, the 'real blot on the system is that the Council has power without responsibility . . . but . . . they understand the importance of things, and are only too glad to say, "We are powerless," when their knowledge of affairs tells them that to act on their prejudices would involve really serious consequences.'[64]

The heavyweights in the India Council during Curzon's time were Sir William Lee-Warner and Sir Alfred Lyall. Since they were old 'India Hands', it was obvious that they would have decided views about the administration of India, which clashed with the Viceroy's. Curzon attributed this to professional jealousy. There were also Sir Charles Crosthwaite, who got on well with Lyall and was, as Lyall was at times, also a keen opponent of Curzon's policies, but a favourite of Godley's,[65] Sir Steuart Bayley and Sir Dennis Fitzpatrick, ex-Lieutenant Governor of the Punjab, whom Curzon singled out as being a keen critic of his policies, in the mould of Sir Lee-Warner, again an eminent old India hand but by no means a Curzon supporter. There was also Sir A. MacDonnell, freshly back from India.

Sir William Lee-Warner is one Councillor whose personality shines through the Council's Minutes as a fierce and public opponent of Curzon's 'centralization' plans. He was a complex man; he did not approve of Kitchener's military reform plans but nevertheless backed his proposal to station three British battalions in India, especially in Western India, which he correctly surmised was the political mainspring of nascent Indian nationalism; on the other hand, Sir I. Finlay objected to this proposal, because the thought that devoting the budget surplus to military expenditure would be less constructive in terms of keeping the Indians happy than announcing a tax revision. Thus, we can reach conclusions about the extent to which the various individual Councillors participated actively in the proceedings and discussions of the Council and to what extent they employed their specialisms to this end.

The person who dissented the most, in fact, was Sir Denis Fitzpatrick, ex-Lieutenant Governor of the Punjab, which rather vindicated Richmond Ritchie's assessment of him as being mired in Punjab politics. He also rather bore out Curzon's assessment that the councillors wanted to keep their hands in on the governance of an India they had left. One especially useful volume is that which details the dissensions made by various councillors over the years.[66] Dissent by a particular councillor of course did not mean that that particular piece of legislation did not go through, in fact, the Minutes of dissent record the views of those opposing legislation that had been passed through. It is in these Minutes that the individualities of the councillors truly shine through, and it is also possible to discern how individual councillors felt about contemporary politics in Asia. From this volume we see that Fitzpatrick was responsible for eleven of the twenty-three non-consensual decisions handed down by the Council of India in Curzon's time, and nine of those related to the Punjab: three pertaining to the Punjab Land Alienation Act, and the other six to the proposed railway expansion of the Frontier—while being ready to acknowledge that the policy of the

Punjab Government had at times been wanting with regard to Frontier administration, Fitzpatrick, nevertheless, could not resist a swipe at Curzon's 'forward' policy, which was resented by those who preferred to train greater focus on securing the internal administration of India, nor did he approve of what he perceived as the Viceroy taking sole control of frontier policy.

Until Sir Hugh Barnes took up his place on the Council, Lyall appears to have been the only one to carry on a regular correspondence with Curzon; not, of course, that the Councillors were obligated to do so, but such would have enabled them to revise and update their knowledge of Indian conditions. Curzon obviously regarded Barnes as a capable administrator, offering him the Governorship of Bombay, but his views, on matters of comprehensive policy direction, were very different from those of the elder statesman. As Lyall wrote to the Viceroy,

> The foreign relations of India are regulated by a kind of unwritten Monroe doctrine . . . we maintain over all the countries immediately adjacent the policy of allowing no intervention by other European nations, and the predominance of no influence except our own. [This] gives us such incessant occupation abroad in Asia, and brings us into continual contact or collision with European rivals.[67]

This was exactly the line taken by most of the British Government, their apprehensions about unleashing Curzon in India revolving around the possible diplomatic fallout with the rest of the world. While Curzon's aggressive imperialism might have reflected the spirit of the age, it did not reflect the spirit of the tottering Conservative Government in the early years of Edward VII. Nor would it endear him to administrative veterans who had come through the Mutiny and did not want to rock the boat again. That Curzon wanted Lyall in India when the latter was known not to support all his ideas is just another illustration of how he did not care about personal compatibility, but merely efficiency, when choosing people.

The others, barring Crosthwaite, do not seem to have roused themselves to write at all, and by 1902 (which was when he declined, for the second time, the offer of Bombay) even Lyall's energies were flagging. As he admitted, 'I am now so near the end of my time [at the India Office] that my interest . . . is languishing.'[68] A Viceroy, especially one of Curzon's energy, could not have been faulted had he construed this as proof that the Councillors only hung on to their seats for pecuniary benefits, not out of any real interest in India. To some extent this was true; the Councillors used their positions to claim prime posts for their families. Both Lyall and Crosthwaite used the Viceroy's intercession to obtain appointments for their sons in India; Crosthwaite in the Central Provinces Commission—and Lyall in the Political Service, incidentally proving that the Councillors were not averse to put in requests for favours from a Viceroy they were allergic to. But Curzon had the pleasure of informing Crosthwaite that clearance for his son's appointment lay with Hamilton; he could comment with ironic satisfaction that, 'I doubt not your colleagues in the India Office will be equally ready with myself to forward the career of the young man.'[69] Lyall's son-in-law was appointed a Secretary to the Viceroy's camp.

It was possibly this desire to retain such undoubtedly advantageous and influential posts, with little attendant consequential responsibility, which engendered the over-cautiousness that Dawkins was quick to scathingly point out to Curzon; as a rule, he said, Lyall 'sees a thing from at least six different points of view, and leaves his hearer to make up his own mind.'[70] The 'delay' this caused in seeing through (or not) legislation was certain to grate on a Viceroy who was convinced of the righteousness of his plans. This indecisiveness of the councillors was well-known to all, and thus it came as a big surprise when they unanimously backed so large-scale a reform as the 'partition' of Bengal; Lawrence wrote to the Viceroy that he had fully expected them to funk it.[71] But, going by the placidly affirmative responses of the India Council to such major legislation, including the Punjab Land Alienation Act, the Police Reforms, and the creation of the NWFP, it is apparent that they reserved

the exercise of their powers for relatively minor reforms. As to the
Council not interfering in major reforms, Curzon remarked that he
relied upon 'that quite invaluable Godley'[72] and the Secretary of State
(at that time George Hamilton) to ensure that this state of affairs
continued. It is contentious as to why the Council should pass major
reforms if they really disliked Curzon's style of administration, unless
they really did not wish to jeopardise the functioning of the Government
of India by their petty squabbles. Nor does it explain why Hamilton
could not exercise his powers in getting the Council to acquiesce in
Curzon's minor reforms as well. Nonetheless, Curzon's claim as to
Hamilton's support is backed up, as we have seen above, by Curzon's
ex-Finance Member and City executive Clinton Dawkins.

And while Curzon was undoubtedly thankful that the Council generally
only 'interfered' in smaller, less important pieces of legislation, he
wondered how that justified their existence, especially when minor
modifications were often made in response to alterations in the local
scene, which the Council would not, obviously, be personally cognisant
of. There was the proposal to relieve the Punjab Government of the
administration of Simla. The Council cavilled. Curzon fumed that he
did not know what the Council existed for, 'if it is to be at liberty to
reject *in toto* a scheme, elaborated by the Government of India with
infinite labour, on so purely a local subject as the future administration
of Simla, put forward by a unanimous [Viceroy's] Council, and
supported by two successive Lieutenant Governors of the Punjab, the
very people who are going to be despoiled.'[73] From this it would appear
that Curzon chiefly thought that the India Council's principal role
should be that of a guiding body providing experience on major issues
of polity using the vast accumulated experience of its members as a
contextual light. It would also appear that he felt it should step in only
when a decision was not fully backed by all those in immediate power
in India, or that it was a likely to raise controversy or people had serious
objections as to its workability. Curzon was, in fact, anxious to reduce
the size of the Council, advocating a paring down by not filling in

vacancies as they arose.[74] His vision for the Council appears to have been that of a broad advisory body, composed of people having latterly returned from India, which would provide for a continuum of policy and a contextual assessment of new legislation as it was introduced, as opposed to long—retired specialists who had made their mark in concentrated areas of polity. When Crosthwaite retired, he rejected a Colonel Yate to fill in the vacancy, because, among other things, the colonel's 'knowledge [was] confined entirely to the frontier and only to certain sections of the frontier.'[75] It is possible that Curzon felt that appointing a person who specialised in a narrow area would merely lead to that individual insisting on his views being carried out over those of the Viceroy's, and inducing the rest of the Council to do the same. It was the argument for the statesman's view of overarching polity as opposed to the bureaucrat's view of narrow administration.

Another Councillor was Sir J. Westland, who took his place on the Council immediately after going home following a stint as the Finance Member on the Viceroy's Council. Curzon had found him an agreeable person to work with, barring that fact that his 'financial puritanism' led him into collisions with the other members of the Viceroy's Council. Possibly this 'Puritanism' continued when Westland became a Councillor on the India Council. He, however, seemed to have an astute politico-economic brain, and over the question of the imposition of sugar duties observed to Curzon that, 'we [the Government of India] are wanted as the stalking horse, from behind whom the Home Government propose to slay an independent quarry.'[76] It would appear that Westland's predecessor as Finance Member, Sir J. Mackay, was similarly non-troublesome, though so tied up in City finance that he did not consider questions from other political angles at all. As Hamilton wrote to Curzon, echoing his private secretary Sir Richmond Ritchie, who would later prove to be a keen sympathiser of Curzon's, Mackay was a 'very able man, influenced by a most intelligent commercial instinct, but his ideas and views are not those of the Council generally. He has none of the *esprit de corps* of the Indian Civil

Service; he is in no sense hampered or influenced by the traditions of that service.'[77] The notation that the Finance Member was not always in tandem with the crusty ways of the rest of the council is all the more interesting when one notes that the Council most asserted its power over the Viceroy in matters financial as opposed to legislative, often citing financial constraints as a reason for turning down Curzon's proposals. In fact, even Hamilton and Godley noted that that the Councillors were usually very happy to endorse any sort of legislative proposal, but were obstructive on most questions of financial legislation. According to Godley this was because blocking finance proposals gave them a chance to demonstrate their power over the incumbent Viceroy, while not standing in the way of better administration which could affect the mindsets of the governed 'in matters in which the public interest seems to them not to be seriously involved, they should be apt to assert their supremacy.'[78] The conscientious Hamilton looked further into this propensity of the India Council and remarked that it did not bide well, as India did not need as much legislation as was then being applied to it (by Curzon) and it would be better for all concerned if the India Council blocked some of that.[79]

In this case there was another aspect to the Council's objections; the funds for expansion looked likely to be drawn from the English Treasury, not the Indian, and it may well have been the possibility of protests from Parliament that made the Council proceed warily.

A more affable Councillor was Sir Steuart Bayley. Like everyone (apart from the Finance Member) on the India Council, Sir Steuart's views had undoubtedly been shaped by his time in the ICS. It was natural that councillors seeking a continuum would view contemporary policies in the light of their own times in India. Bayley's career had followed the classic trajectory of an ICS career, with the additional proviso that he had spent most of his time in Bengal; but it is possible that having served there through the famines of 1872–73, he understood the need for administrative flexibility.[80]

It is thus apparent that the India Council was not a monolithic, homogeneous body whose members stuck up for each other; certainly it would appear that it took new members some time to get into the proper clannish spirit of things! Councillors did not always agree or disagree on the same issue, nor was any one Councillor responsible for trying to block a course of action being decided upon or a directive being issued. There were also conflicts, it is true, between the personal, the political and ideological personae of individuals. People like Hamilton, though officially part of the 'London clique', and even there representing dual offices and interests, sympathised with the Viceroy, even as they valued their positions in an official world not always in tune with Curzon's aspirations. The keynote here was to continually strike and maintain a delicate balance. But it also does not appear that there were power blocks and cliques among the Councillors, pro- and anti-Curzon factions; factions for and against specific lines of polity. Curzon was mistaken, too, when he stated that the Councillors seemed to have deliberately ranged themselves against him. Lee-Warner and Fitzpatrick were both hostile to many of his policies and reforms in India, but they did not collaborate or back each other up in Council to create a block of opinion, something that they could have brought about had they manoeuvred sufficiently.

In fact, by itself, without its head, the Secretary of State, the Council was not autonomous. It was a body whose chief grouse against the Viceroy was alleged over-centralization, and which used powers born of its constitutional superiority to concentrate, i.e., centralize Indian administration in London, but the paradox was illusive; the power over Indian administration thus taken from the Viceroy did not devolve onto the Council, but its head in his capacity as Secretary of State. The problem was the struggle over the 'need to identify the unit of autonomy,'[81] a process, in fact, that could be said to be ongoing with respect to the provinces and the Government of India as well. But this was not as simplistic as deciding whether ultimate power lay with the Government of India or the India Office, because 'the boundaries [of autonomy] are blurred inside the organizations as well as at its boundaries with related organizations.'[82] In terms of immediate constitutional superiority, it was the India Office that had the ultimate veto over any Viceroy's plans; were ultimate paramountcy considered, such veto would lie with the Cabinet.

It was true that, being composed of ex-India Hands, the Council's members would have decisive views on Indian domestic administration, but none of the Councillors in Curzon's time had much experience of foreign policy, on which lay the greatest points of friction between Curzon and the Cabinet. Here, the Council could be vulnerable to political manipulation, persuaded by the Cabinet ministers and the Colonial office that Curzon's moves were potentially damaging to the Imperial fabric. They, or their alleged views- could be used as self-exculpatory justifications for a move endorsed by the Secretary of State which he knew to be unpopular with the Viceroy. In 1904 Brodrick cited the Council's feelings as proof that advancing on Gyantse, the Tibetan city on the road to Lhasa, would be a mistake: 'I have seen individually men differing so much as Sir Steuart Bayley, Sir James Mackay, Sir John Gordon, Sir Charles Crosthwaite . . . they all of them object to advancing.'[83]

The Council could also be used, more blatantly, as a cat's paw. As illustrated above, the Council was often used as a means of justifying the actions of the Secretary of State or Godley. But it could go further; Balfour, wishing to exonerate Brodrick from Curzon's charge that he was obstructive, explained that the Secretary of State was sandwiched between the Council and the Viceroy,[84] overlooking the fact that as Secretary of State Brodrick was head of the Council, with the power to overrule it, and as to the Viceroy, he was his constitutional superior, with the power to overrule him as well. And certainly he enjoyed the support of much of the Council. Curzon was not above using the Council as a tool to wriggle out of diplomatically sticky situations either, writing to Balfour that he had actually wondered whether 'Brodrick's advisers at the India Office,'[85] not Brodrick per se, desired to drive him to resign, thus preserving the modicum of a façade of amiability between himself, the head of the Council, and their Prime Minister.

The India Office's attempts to dictate Indian policy to a Viceroy appointed precisely on account of his specialist knowledge of the Indian Empire met with only partial success. In any case, it was probably ill-advised. As has been noted with regard to the Bombay Government and the many superior governments it was answerable to, the 'job for which the Home Government was best fitted was that of laying down broad principles of policy for the guidance of the Indian authorities. For them to attempt to go further . . . was neither practicable nor politic.'[86] Curzon was not employing hyperbole when he stated that the British Government could not treat the Government of India, as though it were a 'subordinate department', of itself. Constitutionally, the Government of India was not answerable to the Cabinet. The Viceroy was answerable to the Secretary of State, who was appointed by the party in power, but beyond that the link stopped. A Viceroy could not be recalled even if the party he happened to be a member of was kicked out of office in England. He was not bound to follow the doctrines of the ruling party in England. So Curzon's struggles for autonomy from the India Office were much murkier and bitterly fought out than his clashes with anyone else involved in the running of the Indian Empire. This may be attributed mostly to the fact that the India Office was the final arbiter on all India affairs. But it was also because the constituent components of the India Office possessed a greater cohesiveness and integration during the latter half of Curzon's time in office than they ever did at any other time.

Notes

1. Richmond Ritchie, Esq., Pvt. Secretary to Secretary of State for India, writing an assessment of the Councillors on the India Council. Ritchie to Curzon, 23 August 1901, Curzon Papers, Mss Eur F111/160.

2. Curzon to Godley, 27 January 1904, Midleton Papers, Add. Mss. 50072.

3. A.P. Kaminsky, 'The India Office in the Late Nineteenth Century', in *British Imperial Policy: A Reassessment—1858-1912*, N.G. Barrier and Robert I. Crane (eds.), (New Delhi: Heritage Publishers, 1981), p. 27.

4. Ian Copland, 'The Bombay Political Service, 1863–1924', (D.Phil thesis, University of Oxford, 1969), p. 14.

5. George Curzon, *British Government in India: The Story of the Viceroys and Government Houses, Vol. 2*, (London: Cassell & Co., 1925), p. 49.

6. Kaminsky, 'The India Office in the Late Nineteenth Century', in *British Imperial Policy: A Reassessment—1858-1912*, N.G. Barrier and Robert I. Crane (eds.), (New Delhi: Heritage Publishers, 1981), p. 38.

7. Dawkins to Curzon, 17 May 1900, Curzon Papers, Mss Eur F111/181.

8. Godley to Ampthill, 01 July 1904, Ampthill Papers, Mss Eur E233/37.

9. Dawkins to Curzon, 17 May 1900, Curzon Papers, Mss Eur F111/181.

10. Curzon to Balfour, 19 July 1905, Balfour Papers, Add. Mss. 49733.

11. S. Gopal, *British Policy in India 1858-1905*, (London: Cambridge University Press, 1965), p. 222.

12. Kaminsky, *The India Office*, p. 139.

13. Cf. Chapter Four, page XXX [to be added once manuscript is complete].

14. Godley to Lawrence, 18 January 1899, Curzon Papers, Mss Eur F111/181.

15. The explicit use of the term 'British subject' is significant, contrasting as it does with Balfour's satirical comment that if Curzon had his way, India would be raised to the status of an independent and not always friendly power.

16. Curzon to Morley, 17 June 1900, *Curzon Papers*, Mss Eur F111/181.

17. Godley to Curzon, 03 February 1899, Curzon Papers, Mss Eur F111/181.

18. Curzon to Godley, 04 January 1904, extract reproduced in Kilbracken Papers, Mss Eur F102/60.

19. Brodrick to Curzon, 18 May 1905, Midleton Papers, Add. Mss 50077.

20. Arthur Godley, *Reminiscences of Lord Kilbracken*, (London: Macmillan and Co., 1931), p. 198.

21. Godley, *Reminiscences*, pp. 179–80.

22. Godley to Curzon, 1 January 1901, Kilbracken Papers, Mss Eur F102/60.

23. Godley, *Reminiscences*, pp. 179–80.

24. Godley, *Reminiscences*, pp. 182–3.

25. Godley to Curzon, 14 April 1905, Curzon Papers, Mss Eur F111/168.

26. This is a suspicious statement. The letter was written in May 1905, when it was known that Curzon planned to stay on in India for at least another year and come home the following spring. The Partition was to come into effect on 16 August 1905, when Curzon would still have been in India. Did Godley have insider knowledge of any plan that was preconceived to drive the Viceroy into resigning?

27. Godley to Curzon, 30 May 1905, Curzon Papers, Mss Eur F111/168.

28. Curzon to Godley, 03 May 1905, Curzon Papers, Mss Eur F111/168.

29. Godley to Hamilton, 29 July 1902, Hamilton Papers, Mss Eur F123/62.

30. Curzon to Hamilton, 11 May 1905, Curzon Papers, Mss Eur F111/183.

31. Gopal, *British Policy in India*, p. 292.

32. Hamilton to Curzon, 06 November 1902, Mss Eur F111/161.

33. Curzon to Hamilton, 27 November 1902, Mss Eur F111/161.

34. Curzon to Balfour, 20 November 1902, Mss Eur F111/161.

35. Gilmour, *Curzon*, p. 136.

36. Rose, *Superior Person*, pp. 350–1.

37. Ibid., p. 351.

38. Balfour to Curzon, 01 January 1905, Balfour Papers, Add. Mss 49733.

39. Dawkins to Curzon, 06 June 1900, Curzon Papers, Mss Eur F111/181.

40. Dawkins to Curzon, 06 June 1900, Curzon Papers, Mss Eur F111/181.

41. William St. John Midleton, *Records and Recollections*, (London: John Murray, 1939), p. 198.

42. Knollys to Sandars, 09 September 1905, Balfour Papers, Vol 3, in Young, *Balfour: The Happy Life*, p. 241.

43. Balfour to the King, 19 July 2005, Balfour Papers, Vol. 3, cited in Young, *Balfour*, p. 240.

44. Brodrick to Curzon, 29 October 1903, Midleton Papers, 22/3.

45. Curzon to Brodrick, 02 October 1903, Midleton Papers, 22/3.

46. Balfour to Curzon, 09 June 1905, Balfour Papers, Add. Mss 49733.

47. Brodrick to Knollys, 04 September 1905, Midleton Papers, Add. 50072.

48. Balfour to Knollys, 07 October 1905, Midleton Papers, Add. 50072.

49. This is not a snide comment on the abilities of the ICS, but rather a reflection of the fact that no ICS man, apart from Lawrence, was ever appointed Viceroy of India, given that they were mostly not of titled descent.

50. Barnes to Curzon, 04 August 1905, Curzon Papers, Mss Eur F111/183.

51. Curzon to Brodrick, 12 January 1905, Midleton Papers, Add. Mss 50077.

52. Dawkins to Curzon, 17 May 1900, Curzon Papers, Mss Eur F111/181.

53. The following Councillors actually occupied office at some point or other during Curzon's Viceroyalty: Gen. Sir D.M. Stewart, 1885–1900; Sir J.B. Peile, 1887–1902; Sir A.C. Lyall, 1888–1903; Sir Charles H.T. Crosthwaite, 1895–1905; Sir Steuart C. Bayley, 1895–1905; F.C. Le Merchant, 1896–1906; Sir Dennis Fitzpatrick, 1897–1907; Sir J.J. Mackay, 1897–1911; Sir P.P. Hutchins, 1898–1908; Sir James Westland, 1899–1903; Lieut.-Gen. A.B. Babcock, 1901–07; Sir William Lee-Warner, 1902–12; Sir A.P. MacDonnell, 1903–05; I.F. Finlay, 1903–06; Sir Hugh Barnes, 1905–13.

54. See below.

55. For an illustration see Kaminsky, *The India Office*, pp. 46–7.

56. Dawkins to Curzon, 24 May 1900, Curzon Papers, Mss Eur F111/181.

57. St. John Brodrick, *Relations of Lord Curzon as Viceroy of India with the British Government, 1902–5*, (London: n.p. May 1926), p. 2, Mss Eur B189.

58. Sir Alfred Lyall cited in Sir Mortimer Durand, *Life of the Right Hon. Sir Alfred Comyn Lyall*, (Edinburgh/London: William Blackwood & Sons, 1913), p. 327.

59. Curzon to Brodrick, 02 March 1905, Curzon Papers, Mss Eur F111/168.

60. Brodrick to Ampthill, 10 June 1904, Ampthill Papers, Mss Eur E233/37.

61. Godley, *Reminiscences*, p. 164.

62. Clinton Dawkins to Curzon, 19 December 1901, Curzon Papers, Mss Eur F11/182.

63. Godley to Curzon, 03 February 1899, Curzon Papers, Mss Eur F111/181.

64. Richmond Ritchie to Curzon, 23 August 1901, Curzon Papers, Mss Eur F111/160.

65. Godley to Curzon, 03 March 1905, Curzon Papers, Mss Eur F111/168.

66. Minutes of Dissent by Members of the Council of India, IOR/C/131–132. Also IOR/C/129.

67. Lyall to Curzon, 01 May 1903, cited in Durand, *Life of Sir Alfred Comyn Lyall*, p. 398.

68. Lyall to Curzon, 11 July 1902, Curzon Papers, Mss Eur F111/182.

69. Curzon to Crosthwaite, 19 February 1902, Curzon Papers, Mss Eur F111/182.

70. Dawkins to Curzon, 10 May 1905, Curzon Papers, Mss Eur F1·11/183.

71. Lawrence to Curzon, 05 June 1905, Curzon Papers, Mss Eur F111/183.

72. Curzon to Dawkins, 12 June 1900, Curzon Papers, Mss Eur F111/181.

73. Curzon to Barnes, 14 August 1905, Curzon Papers, Mss Eur F111/183.

74. Curzon to Godley, 23 March 1905, Curzon Papers, Mss Eur F111/168.

75. Curzon to Brodrick, 30 March 1905, Midleton Papers, Add. Mss 50077.

76. Curzon to Godley, 23 February 1899, Curzon Papers, Mss Eur F111/181.

77. Hamilton to Curzon, 14 February 1901, Curzon Papers, Mss Eur F111/160.

78. Godley to Curzon, 14 February 1901, Curzon Papers, Mss Eur F111/160

79. Hamilton to Curzon, 14 February 1901, Curzon Papers, Mss Eur F111/160.

80. See, for example, Raj Jogeshur Mitter, *Biography of Sir Steuart Bayley, K.C.S.I*, (Calcutta: S.K. Lahiri & Co., 1891).

81. Michael Z. Brooke, *Centralization and Autonomy: A Study in Organisational Behaviour*, (London: Holt, Rinehart & Winston, 1984), p. 314.

82. Ibid.

83. Brodrick to Curzon, 06 November 1903, Midleton Papers, 22/3.

84. Balfour to Curzon, 23 August 1905, Balfour Papers, Add. Mss 49733.

85. Curzon to Balfour, 21 September 1905, Balfour Papers, Add. Mss 49733.

86. Copland, 'The Bombay Political Service, 1863–1929', Ch. 3, p. 15.

3

The Ordering of Subordination in the Presidencies

If you have no objection, and if it would not be a bother to you . . . I should like to go to Bombay and bid you Godspeed. I should not . . . cause any official inconvenience as I should go to the Taj Mahal Hotel, and particularly ask that I might be allowed to come and go *without any ceremonial attentions* . . .[1] (emphasis added)

Baron Ampthill to Curzon,
05 September 1905

British India was not the product of a hegemonic drive of conquest. The disparate provinces slipping from Mughal grasp had been conquered by a combination of British and Indian armies from three different bases; Calcutta, Bombay and Madras. While the act of 1858 unified the three 'capitals', the rivalry still smouldered—Bombay in particular—chafing against the reins imposed on its autonomy by Simla.

This chapter seeks to elaborate on the often hinted at, but never regarded as much more than the product of imperialist political gamesmanship, tensions between the Government of India and the Governors of its major presidencies, Bombay and Madras. These tensions rose to the fore during Curzon's Viceroyalty, in part because of his own decided views on the provincial contract and the personal fitness of the incumbent Governors. Further, as explored in the preceding chapter, Curzon's Viceroyalty marked an apex in political intrigue within the India Office, and the Governors of Bombay and Madras, being senior administrators handpicked by the India Office, were understandably drawn into the fray. Finally, because Curzon was the first Viceroy to install a Governor as *locum temens* while he went on leave, it meant that there was a good deal more procedural upheaval than there had ever been before.

Curzon often complained about his Governors and Lieutenant Governors being non-entities, and the scarcity of monographs about them do not appear to provide evidence to the contrary. Even as historians rail against centralization and the cult of personality in British India, their output is evidence of their own contribution to making this form of historiography dominant over all others.

THE SIMLA–BOMBAY–MADRAS STATUS QUO

The obstacles to a smooth relationship between Curzon and the Governors started with the mode of selecting the governors themselves. The Governors of Bombay and Madras, like the Viceroy, were appointed by the Crown for a term of five years, and were usually from the aristocracy. Given the half-way house status of these Governorships— being the headships of provinces of British India, they did not confer the same prestige or powers upon the incumbent as a pro-consular post would—it was difficult to find suitable personages, and the appointments often degenerated into 'society appointments'. Because the Governor did not normally have specific Indian experience, he had a Council consisting of a team of two members (as opposed to the Viceroy's six-man Council) of the Indian Civil Service of twelve years' standing to assist him from that particular presidency's secretariat. This, as Curzon perceived, was the major flaw in a system where the Governors tended to be parachuted in from the outside: it made them susceptible to the depredations of the Bombay or Madras cadres. Finally, the Presidency Governor possessed the privilege of communicating directly with the Secretary of State,[2] which put him in a position to carry objections about the Viceroy directly to the Viceroy's constitutional superior. The Governors themselves treasured this mark of distinction because it was not open to the heads of other presidencies and provinces, and they considered that it elevated Bombay and Madras to a higher status by comparison. None of this was acceptable to Curzon, who wanted uniformity in administration, and did not like grey areas, or those that could be considered as such.

Thus, on the surface, the extant status quo looks simplistic; an authoritarian Viceroy backed by his status as head of the Government of India in India seeking to co-opt recalcitrant subordinates into a system of deference to Simla. But there are dualistic themes and angles to this; the individual governors and/versus the 'temper' of the presidency; at times converging and at times diverging. In the case of the Bombay and Madras Presidencies it was not only a power tussle between the Centre and the State, such as that which convolutes India today. It was also rife with questions of personal and institutional rivalry. In some cases there might be a disagreement with the Governor over issues of personal prestige (as in the case of Ampthill who shared Curzon's penchant for ceremonial grandeur he thought would befit his position) while the administrative side would meet with Viceregal approval, as was also the case with Ampthill. On the other hand, the Viceroy (and perhaps the incumbent Governor) would come up against the inherent work culture of a particular presidency, while approving of the Governor. Thus, there were even differences in the approach with which the Presidencies and their Governors sought to negotiate away their 'subordinate to Simla' status. The only base commonality between both Bombay and Madras was that even as the 'independent' Governors were often backed by Whitehall in their quest for greater autonomy (or, more precisely, the Viceroy attracted censure for not being gentle with them), ultimately, they were constitutionally subordinate to the Government of India, and so were their presidencies. Their subordinate position was pre-ordained; what remained were the struggles over reducing this subordination to a mere constitutionalism (or not) against the backdrop of an inchoate realisation of the existence of a pan-Indian landscape.

Diagram 1

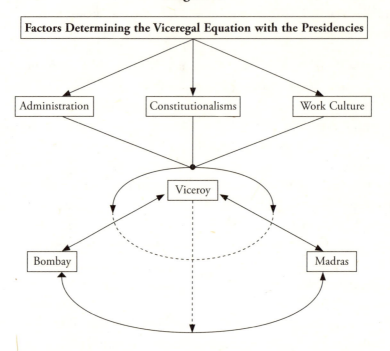

Diagrammatically, the framework of the Curzon–Bombay–Madras relationships may be expressed as above. As apparent from the diagram, the following operative factors were instrumental in determining the nature of the Viceroy's two-way relationship with the Governors of both Bombay and Madras: Administration, Constitutionalisms, and Work Cultures. These, channelled through the personality of the incumbent Viceroy and expressed to the Governors, then acquired their peculiar characteristics when perceived by diverse individual Viceroys and Governors. In its turn, the Viceregal relationship (or the perception of it) with one of the given Presidencies set the tone for inter-presidency relationships between Bombay and Madras.

It will thus be apparent that there were many rivalries contained within the apparently uni-dimensional Simla–Presidencies equations. This chapter will analyse the main threads of contention and differences, and examine how they manifested themselves under Curzon and the various

Governors who served under him: Sandhurst,[3] Northcote,[4] and Lamington[5] in Bombay; Havelock and Ampthill in Madras. These relationships would have been rendered complex because of the traditional friction between these two presidencies and Calcutta, and also because these were political appointments and the appointees, one would assume, possessed a degree of intriguing clout in the close-knit governing circles of late Victorian England. Plus they turned out to be not very capable administrators, except, apparently, Ampthill, and Northcote.

Against this, in the following chapter, will be set Curzon's apparently unproblematic relationship with the Lieutenant Governor of the United Provinces, and his stormy relationship with the Lieutenant Governor of the Punjab. This chapter will also illustrate how Curzon's relationship with Ampthill,[6] the Governor of Madras who was his locum as Acting Viceroy, got off to a bad start but matured into one of professional respect. Curzon's relationship with the Second Baron Ampthill is a central case study, as Ampthill was Governor of Madras for all of Curzon's Viceroyalty and also acting Viceroy when Curzon went Home on leave in 1904. It will then focus on the Viceroy's less intense engagement with the Governors of the Bombay Presidency (as opposed to his administrative work in the same presidency) as a means to highlight the flaws in the functioning of the administration of these two presidencies.

The major sources will be the private papers of the major figureheads, specifically the sections which contain their official correspondence with each other, my contention being that there is much to be revealed in the language of diplomacy. Rather than picking out myself the anecdotes and evidences which are symptomatic of the prickly Simla–Bombay–Madras relationship, this thesis will use the incidences that seem to have inflamed the principal participants most and been construed by them as being slights from their central or provincial counterparts.

The core, overarching, unifying theme in the power struggle between the Centre and the Presidencies was Centralization, in principle and as it impinged upon administrative affairs (this would have affected Bombay more) and the expression of decentralization and provincial autonomy in the presidencies' ceremonial trappings (which Madras, or its incumbent Governors, seemed to feel the greater).

CENTRALIZATION VS. DECENTRALIZATION: THE CORE OF THE CONFLICT

Curzon once remarked on the Madras Governor's probable reaction if one of his districts came to him and demanded the same independence he saw Madras to be demanding vis-à-vis the Government of India.[7] This comment, startlingly foreshadowing Midleton's that if Curzon had his way, India would be raised to the status of an independent and not always friendly power vis-à-vis the Government of Britain, reveals the deep-rooted belief in adhering to established hierarchies of power within the governmental corpus of the Indian Empire. Centralization (and its opposite) was always going to remain a relative term; this does not, however, mean that the people fighting for or against it saw it in such dispassionate lights.

Centralization essentially amounted to a concentration, as opposed to a federalized, diffusion of power. For Bombay and Madras, however, the resistance to centralization was as much due to the nature of the centralization and the administrative spheres it affected as the principle of the thing, apart from the loss of control over their administrations. Pre-Curzonian decentralization meant that administrative matters in Bombay and Madras were more often dealt with internally, and thus did not come to the forefront in their dealings with Simla. The combination of Curzon's exactitude and his 'centralizing' zeal ensured that their affairs were now at the forefront of Viceregal scrutiny.

There were, basically, two arms to the centralization debate: financial and administrative, the latter affecting, or having the potential to affect, the provinces' control over their finances. Both Bombay and Madras were only partially in control of their financial commitments, the regulations for which were decided every five years when the proportional distributions between the Centre and the various provinces of India was worked out in a formula known as the Provincial Contract.[8] It would appear that Bombay and Madras felt that if centralization was to be imposed, then their financial expenses should be borne by Simla in greater proportion (cf. the Municipal boards row). In the case of Madras, Havelock, especially virulent about the perceived ill-effects of centralization, focussed largely on the financial, whereas his successor, whose administration was certainly better than Havelock's, was concerned with administrative autonomy. The prime concern of the Presidencies, especially Madras, as to over-centralization centred around its financial drawbacks to themselves, which was why they argued for financial decentralization. But Curzon's prime concerns as regards centralization or otherwise were centred around issues of legislative and administrative autonomy. As he explained to Havelock,

> When we have been writing about over-centralization . . . we have had in our minds rather different things. Your eye has been fixed throughout on the Provincial Contract . . . [but] it is a matter of correspondence between our Governments. . . . I do not know that I am particularly enamoured of the Provincial Contract system.[9]

What Curzon meant by centralization was that the presidency governments and Simla could engage together on legislative issues; he did not want the Central Government to be seen as merely an issuer of laws or a government that was a rubber stamp to provincial decisions.

In the realm of internal administration, an issue that affected both Presidencies, it was the lack of financial autonomy that prompted an outcry. Ampthill had enjoined the newly appointed Lamington to read the *Life* of Sir Bartle Frere, the legendary 1860s Governor of Bombay, as an example of the argument against centralization.[10] Frere, who was steeped in the lore of the Bombay Presidency, having started his career at Poona, eventually rose to be one of the most efficient Governors of Bombay. To illustrate the ludicrousness of the tendency to centralization, his biographer states that, as a result of it, 'the Bombay Government was not even left to reform and organise its own Public Works Department (in Frere's day the PWD made some wholesale changes, such as finally destroying the battlements of the old Bombay Fort), but was forced to make it conform to the Calcutta Secretary's notions of what was best.'[11] Such an argument against centralization was a conflation of the defence of 'ancient privilege', the virtues of the man on the spot, and the inability of the Government of India to control and manage a highly centralized structure. Indeed Frere's biographer claimed that even a Viceroy's powers were eroded as a result of centralization (Curzon's motive for the same being quite the reverse) claiming that, 'the departments at Calcutta become more and more independent, each secretary administering his own with less and less consultation with his colleagues or the Governor General, who often knew little of what was being done till he was appealed to put an end to friction or settle a farce.'[12] This sentiment, if quite in a different context, was echoed by Curzon.

Decentralization for the Bombay Government did not extend to financial self-sufficiency. It is also notable that only 1.86 lac rupees of the famine relief expenditure made by the Bombay Government came from a combination of local government and charitable funds.[13] This would suggest that famine relief was exclusively the prerogative of the centre; the presidencies were quite happy to have access to centrally managed funds. Like Bombay, Madras also chafed at its relative lack of autonomy in financial matters.[14] Prudently, such dissent was directed to Hamilton, who might be safely relied upon to communicate it to Curzon, who would probably furnish a stinging, if accurate reply, if the Governor suggested it to him. There was some truth in Madras' argument. He seemed to feel that with increasing legislative autonomy, the provincial governments would increasingly 'treat the supreme Government [i.e., the Government of India] as though they were merely a post office for the transmission of their correspondence to the Secretary of State.'[15] In this particular case the Madras Government had wanted the Viceroy to ask the Secretary of State to endorse a punitive police force for disturbed districts in South India (possibly Tinnelvely); they did not ask for the Viceroy or the Indian Police Commission's opinion, and did not go into the financial specifics either. There are interesting nuances to this episode. First of all it would appear that the provincial governments had a very good idea as to the exact delimitations of a Viceroy's power, especially in relation to London. It is also interesting that Havelock did not use his own right of correspondence with the Secretary of State to forward his plea, but went via the Viceroy, which would seem to be an acknowledgement of a Viceroy's supremacy in India. It is also possibly a realization of the fact that Hamilton would not have taken kindly to an administrative request which came to him over the head of the Viceroy. In effect, Madras was using the Viceroy's constitutional superiority as a means of getting what they wanted, and also remaining in the Viceroy's good books by a seeming subservience to that authority.[16]

But Curzon took pride in micro-managing local governments from Simla; such centralizing was, of course, the best way of ensuring that the macro-reforms he was instituting contained any appliqué value at all and percolated down the Presidential Governments, thus, coming into contact with the daily lives of 'the Governed', who were, of course, to be kept happy if the Empire was to remain stable. This would explain the reason why even the relatively non-important Madras Municipal Corporation (Bombay being responsible for a mercantile empire and Calcutta being the seat of Government) faced Curzon's reforming zeitgeist. This too was tied up with centralization and provincial responsibility for their own finances; the Madras Board objected to having a grant of 150,000 rupees converted into a loan.[17] They argued that since, at Home, Imperial aid was granted to local resources, the same principle should be applied in India. In this case, of course, they appeared very willing to acknowledge their subordination to the Government of India. Over finances, thus, the issue of who would wield overall authority was compromised over ideals of economy.

Not unnaturally, the Governors of Madras and Bombay threw themselves into the campaign against centralization. Havelock[18] told Curzon that,

> holding as I do very strongly these views on the need for further decentralization. . . . I cannot agree . . . that the presidential Governments are already in some ways independent. Possibly, if I were Viceroy, I might think as you do in this matter, but being Governor of Madras, I cannot.[19]

However, even when his successor as Governor, the Second Baron Ampthill, became acting Viceroy in 1904, he certainly did not use the opportunity to 'see the matter as Curzon did,' but contrarily, straightway reassured his Bombay counterpart of his enduring commitment to decentralization.[20] The other grievance Ampthill did not hesitate to raise straightaway, in the same letter, was that of the Bombay and Madras Presidencies' antagonism to 'centralization' [sic]. This would definitely have vindicated Curzon's view that the Governors of these presidencies were incapable of seeing beyond their own small spheres of influence.

> Decentralization [sic] is all very well; but it appears to me, in the case of Bombay and Madras, to have been carried to a point in which the supreme government is nowhere, and of which the petty kings of those dominions are even unconscious that responsibility attaches to anyone but themselves . . . the system seems to me in very urgent need of reform.[21]

He railed against the 'mock independence'[22] claimed by Bombay, telling Godley that 'decentralize as much as you like as regards administrative detail, but not as regards supreme executive authority.'[23]

From the point of view that decreed a Viceroy should be the undisputed executive of the Government of India, Curzon was justified in railing against decentralization. Sometimes decentralization, (especially coupled with un-coordinated appointments) could become a very real impediment to a Viceroy's exercise of free authority. James Fergusson, the Bombay Governor so famously sent out as a backup to the Conservative Lytton, who found himself serving under the Liberal Ripon after election reverses at home, became a real impediment to the reformist Ripon, partly because of his ability to correspond directly with the Secretary of State.[24] Certainly such a complex situation did not arise in the Presidencies during Curzon's Viceroyalty, which marked the apex of the long Conservative ascendancy in British politics.

It would seem, however, that most people at the top of the governmental hierarchy, except Curzon, did not believe centralization to be a good thing insofar as a heterogeneous country like India was concerned. The Home Government, for one, especially after 1903, when Curzon's old friends Balfour and Brodrick were Prime Minister and Secretary of State respectively, seemed to view decentralization as a means of keeping a check on the incumbent Viceroy through manipulation of his Presidency Governors and prominent people from presidency secretariats. The first 'Indian' function St. John Brodrick chaired after becoming Secretary of State in 1904 was a lecture about the Bombay Presidency given by Sir William Lee-Warner at the Society of the Arts in London. Lee-Warner's views, gleaned from long experience in Indian administration, happily coincided with the Home Government's and were also a useful counteraction to the Viceroy's.[25] According to Sir George Birdwood, who was present, the lecture was a direct call for the 'maintenance of the status of [Bombay Presidency's] Administration in having direct dealings with the Secretary of State, as a check upon the centralizing tendencies of the day.' Lee-Warner further said that the Governor of Bombay should be selected by the Crown, because it not only provided India with a statesman in the confidence of the Government, (who could also become Viceroy in Emergencies!) but imposed a check on the 'dangerous tendency of over centralization, by placing Home authorities in direct communication with the Governors.' This was basically encouraging the Governors to sneak on any 'centralization-minded' Viceroy. This in spite of the fact of the three greatest of the Bombay Governors: Frere, Temple, and Elphinstone having been ICS men. The virtues of the 'man on the spot' were also trotted out, but had this principle been stretched to its fullest extent, the 'man on the spot' would logically have risen, like Lawrence, through the ICS. But the Home Government seemed to understand it as 'their man on the spot!' But Lee-Warner's reasoning was that the Government of India is not intended by Parliament to administer the whole Empire, but is charged with control and supervision over all its parts; it is well that it should be able to compare the effects of different systems.'[26]

Others inveighed against centralization from rather more altruistic motives. A curious passage in George Hamilton's memoirs blames Curzon's methods of single-handed reform for aggravating the evil of centralization, which he then proceeds to claim as the cause of the recent upsurge in demands for provincial Home Rule. He then goes on to laud Curzon for sending in his resignation as Viceroy, 'because he had sense enough to see that a similar centralization [presumably to what he assumed Curzon was trying to achieve in civil administration] in military affairs could only result . . . in inefficiency and failure.'[27] This statement of course was made with the hindsight of Kitchener's failure in India, and had not occurred to Hamilton, or anyone else, in 1905.

In 1900, however, Curzon still held the reins, and the formation of the NWFP[28] was another attack on decentralization; a raid near Kohat was brought to the Viceroy's notice nine months after it had occurred. When Curzon wrote to Mackworth Young about this, the Lieutenant Governor, in a fashion similar to that practised by Madras and Bombay, replied that the fault was not his but that of his Secretariat, 'but did you ever hear of such a defence or of such a system?'[29] It might have been said of the defence of their 'ancient privileges' by Bombay and Madras too. It is easy to see how Ampthill became a good administrator once removed from a provincial administration.

Curzon also very astutely turned the tables on those who opposed centralization while hammering out the creation of the NWFP, primarily because the Punjab provincial administration could not cope with the different conditions of governance the frontier required. As he noted, it has frequently been argued that the intervention of a Local Government between the Government of India and the frontier, involves a wise and necessary decentralization . . . on the contrary, it results in centralization of the pettiest and most exasperating description . . . it has yet been the source of exaggerated centralization [and] of interminable delay.[30]

Nor did Curzon miss the point that centralization meant that the Viceroy could assume greater responsibility, with his acknowledged genius for administration, he could only see this as a good thing: 'Of course the Government of India has,' he wrote to Mackworth Young,

from time to time, to overrule all the Local Governments. In a case like that of the Punjab Government the responsibility is largely personal to myself, because the matters concerned ordinarily fall within the scope of the Foreign Department, and relate . . . to Frontier Policy.

By implication, severing the administrative link between the Punjab and the Frontier by the creation of a new Frontier province, would not only free the Punjab government of the irritation caused by the sharing of power, but also mean that frontier concerns would cease to have influence on Punjab legislation and administration. Curzon further stated that such overruling was 'the price that any Lieutenant Governor of the Punjab has to pay for a Viceroy who knows something of the Frontier.'[31] The implication, of course, was that subjects crucial to imperial security could not possibly be left to a mere provincial administration. The only reason that Bombay, even with all its overseas and princely possessions, was not subjected to such stripping was that these charges were not, in Curzon's time, of Imperial concern, i.e., a security threat to Empire, which was possibly a factor that allowed the persistence of Bombay's defiant stance regarding the Government of India—Bombay was not *a priori*. And while Curzon and the Mackworth Youngs[32] totally severed relations with each other over the NWFP episode, it is notable that any bad blood between Curzon and the Presidency Governors was always confined to office. It is thus apparent that Curzon did not always resent his subordinates' attempts to redress his often tactless exercise of righteous power; what he resented was being corrected by an inferior. Bombay and Madras were accorded the status of equal sparring partners, at least in terms of status relative to the other provinces—Curzon himself was not immune to using status as a determinant to interacting with his officials in India.

Apart from the centralization debate, which was properly germane to the issue of executive control of the administration of India, contretemps flared up between Curzon and the Governors over symbolic issues, the main ones being the Governors' constitutionally enshrined right to write to the Secretary of State, and their self-arrogated privilege of having the state bands play the National Anthem for them—both of which Curzon considered to properly belong solely to the Viceroy.

Curzon's objections to the Governors writing directly to the Secretary of State, for one, may be seen as part of his drive to consolidate and extend the under-threat authoritarianism of the Viceroy, especially in the face of 'modern' means of communication. The Governors' aversions to this were simply the result of not wanting to interfere with long established practice. Curzon, it would appear, did not only want to centralize, he wanted to make the Viceregal office a focal point of this centralization. In not underestimating Indian reverence for a strong office and the importance of the existence of some form of supreme authority on the spot in India, he was probably right. But this was not the direction the Home Government wanted, and nor was it the direction an increasingly regionally aware India wanted.

In fact, the Governors appeared to think that Curzon's sole reason for keeping a watchful eye on the administrations of Bombay and Madras was the desire to rob them of their special rights at an opportune moment. 'I can only,' wrote Lamington, 'ascribe the resentment of the Simla Secretariat to the wish to curtail the Madras and B[om]bay Gov[ernmen]ts of . . . their few peculiar privileges.'[33] That he specifically referred to the Secretariat as opposed to the more personalized term 'Viceroy' is perhaps an indication that it was the Bombay cadre as a whole who worried about being supplanted by those lucky enough to get permanent appointments at Simla.

In this case Curzon was probably right in recommending that political appointments to the Governorships of Bombay and Madras be abolished, because they only helped the furtherance of the autonomy these presidencies arrogated to themselves. Taking into account all this, plus the 9th Lancers incident, and his views about the House of Lords, it emerges that Curzon was not at all the pro-aristocratic Tory he is purported to be. In any case, with the exception of MacDonnell, it was the senior ICS officers who appear to have had more active say in matters of administration than provincial governors, or at least (in Madras and Bombay) lobbied actively for suc; and MacDonnell himself had risen through the ranks of the civil service to become Governor of the United Provinces.

MADRAS: GOVERNORS' HAVEN

If centralization was a binding issue of concern for both Bombay and Madras as far as their views on their relationship to Simla were concerned, there were other, unique concerns, as well as subtle differences in the battle against centralization in each of these presidencies. This section looks at Madras.

Madras was far away from the centre of political and commercial action, and politically un-awakened compared to the rest of India. While the shooting of Rand and Ayerst in Bombay in 1897 did not come as a surprise in principle, Havelock had occasion to write to Curzon when the Queen's statue was tarred on her eightieth birthday that he was 'particularly sorry that such a thing should have happened in Madras, a place hitherto conspicuous for immunity from disgraceful acts of this kind.[34] In fact one of Havelock's excuses for not writing to Curzon as frequently as the Viceroy would have liked was that, 'as a rule there is not much to report from this ordinarily tranquil and well-ordered Presidency.'[35]

This Havelock was Sir Arthur Elibank, who probably resented a new Viceroy telling him how to run a province he had been Governor of since 1895. Havelock was perhaps the most intransigent of all the Governors, and his frictional relationship with Curzon seems to have become the historian's basis for claiming rockiness in Curzon's other relationships as well. The Havelock–Curzon correspondence is acrimonious, and singularly graceless in tone as compared to those exchanged between Curzon and Ampthill, Curzon and Lamington, Ampthill and Lamington. They plunge right into business matters rather than dilating on the normative pleasantries usually exchanged between such correspondents. Initially, however, in a stark contrast to the gloomy apprehension with which he viewed Ampthill's appointment, Curzon had been uncritical of the bridge-baptising Sir Arthur,[36] who did indeed have his redeeming features. Curzon strait-jacketed him as 'a type of official whom the Colonial Office turns out,'[37] and later admitted, again to Hamilton, that he had been less than just and that he had found Havelock to be 'quite indifferent to the prejudices of the Indian official . . . hold [ing] just and liberal views about the way in which to administer his province.'[38]

Yet six months later he was fulminating that Havelock was a 'capable controversialist'[39] he had not approved of aspects of the Governors' correspondence with Hamilton, which apparently tended to assume a self-righteous tone. As a matter of fact Havelock seems to have turned the tables very neatly on the Centre, accusing them of proliferating the very thing the Viceroy was attempting to stamp out, i.e., paperwork. An obviously impressed Hamilton included an extract from one of the Governors' letters, infuriating the Viceroy. Havelock complained that,

> as long as circumlocution and centralization have their throne and court at Calcutta and Simla, it is hopeless to expect that the minor administrations, which model themselves upon and love to reflect the glories of the Supreme Government, will change the traditions and practices in which they have been bred.[40]

In the same letter he also stated pompously that another reason for not writing to Curzon (Curzon expected, and returned, a monthly letter from each of his Governors) was that he wrote every week to the Secretary of State, adding in parenthesis that the Governors of Madras and Bombay were required to do this[41] (cf. Lawrence's comment on Old India Hands' resentment of the arrival of the new superior Viceroy) presumably this excused them from writing to their immediate superior. Basically as a governor Havelock was efficient, even as he appears to have adopted a laissez-faire style of administration, especially proving himself in relief operations. In fact, he seems to have been as incensed by administrative inefficiency as his Viceroy; he wrote to Curzon that when he had first arrived in Madras, he had been 'appalled' at the inefficiency of its administration, but having been there for three years, he suggested that he might perhaps have succumbed to the 'Oriental environment',[42] and imbibed something of the Madras cadre's inefficiency. His letters contain many references to the princes of Arcot, Travancore and the Carnatic. He reserved his ire for these princes on the grounds that they were somewhat indifferent administrators, a point which Curzon also worked to eradicate. Hamilton wrote to Curzon almost a year after Havelock's departure that his methods of plague control were being 'universally adopted by the different local administrations . . . he seems [to have struck] the balance between harshness and lavish expenditure.'[43] This, along with the track record of Havelock's successor Ampthill, would prove that however self-important Madras might be, in matters of administration the Presidency seems to have had a humanitarian tradition of administration.

Havelock in fact took an active interest in his successor and appointments to his staff, if only to groom the said successor into upholding Madras' autonomy. One of the papers he left behind for his successor to pursue was a missive composed by member of the Madras Civil Service, outlining the special privileges the Governors of Madras and Bombay were entitled to enjoy in comparison to the lesser Lieutenant Governors of the other provinces. Ampthill duly sent this off as a backing to his own arguments in Madras' favour to the Secretary of State.[44] It is possible that Ampthill's early stormy relationship with Curzon was due to his following Havelock's tradition of administration; as he found his own feet, the relationship proportionately mellowed. The contretemps remained, but took on a more 'Ampthillian character', being flare-ups over ritual as over administrative details, in which Ampthill seems to have been impressed by Curzon's line and applied it efficiently to Madras.

In the cases of Madras, as with the princely states, power struggles were apparently more about the symbols of ritualism, precedence and constitutional status. Precedence was the most fiercely contested, it being the most visible symbol and affirmation of 'superiority' or otherwise. This seems to have been especially aggravated in the case of the Second Baron Ampthill, Governor of Madras from 1900 to1906. Curzon had welcomed the appointment of Ampthill, if with certain misgivings as to how his youth (he was twenty-nine, but had done a stint at the colonial office prior to Madras) would be received by the Madras cadre, and even forewarned Ampthill about the traditional friction between the Madras Government and the Government of India,[45] probably in an attempt to forestall a repetition with himself and Ampthill. But very soon the relationship seems to have degenerated into a worse one (if only temporarily; Curzon later got on capitally with Ampthill, even though he never expressed the very vocal admiration for his administrative prowess that he did for MacDonnell's) than Curzon had with his predecessor Sir Arthur Havelock. Curzon opened with a broadside on the unconstitutionality of Ampthill wishing that the title of 'Her Excellency' be attached to his wife, whereas Curzon wished to reserve the use of this solely for the Vicereine as a mark of her constitutional status.[46] A few posts later, he complained about Ampthill breaking the Indian Warrant of Precedence and giving his sisters-in-law rank over Indian dignitaries,[47] following this up with the charge that the Governor ought not be allowed to have his band play the National Anthem at his approach, because local governors were not entitled to this, because 'the

Governors do not act on behalf of the Sovereign.' Only the Viceroy, representing the Monarch, was entitled to the National Anthem, but the governors of Bombay and Madras insisted, and Havelock had got around the rule by,

> carrying his own band about with him everywhere, and making them play the National Anthem whenever he turned up . . . Ampthill . . . must have it twice. A British regiment plays 'the King' as he approaches the hall; his own band strikes up as he enters it. This . . . is an expansion of ceremonial to which even the Viceroy never aspires.[48]

For Curzon thus, two issues rankled; the unconstitutional practice of playing an anthem whose honour he felt derived from what it represented, and the fact that, by laying greater stress on this form of ceremonial than the Viceroy, the Governors were trying to exalt themselves not only above their stations, but also above that of their constitutional superior, the Viceroy.

The Secretary of State, though 'very desirous of not stirring up this class of question,' fully agreed with Curzon, and replied that he would point this out to Ampthill.[49] But apparently the system continued once Hamilton departed from office, and his successor, St. John Brodrick, did not want to stir up the issue, knowing it to be a sore point with the Bombay and Madras governments, and opined to Curzon that it was 'better to let sleeping dogs lie.'[50] But it was a sore point with Curzon also, and he wrote back acrimoniously that he expected a course of action endorsed by Hamilton to be continually enforced by his successor, and that it should not be left to him to uphold these constitutionalisms of protocol in India: 'it is not for the Viceroy to have friction with his subordinate Governors by rubbing in the orders of the India Office. It is rather for the Secretary of State . . . to remind the offender . . . not to repeat the transgression.'[51] It is apparent that the hierarchy of the Raj was not just based on gradations of power, but also upon specific types of power being exercised by persons in specific offices. To exercise power that was not the general provenance of one's office was itself an indication of possible lack of power or ability to enforce righteous power within that office.

Further, the India Office's lackadaisical response to an issue that was clearly felt deeply by all the Indian administrators involved suggests that they did not grasp the depths the issue sounded in India. One may compare to this their hysterical response when Curzon appealed to the King, over their heads, and thus, according to them, unconstitutionally, to let him announce a tax remission at the Durbar. Then, it was Curzon who was bewildered by the vehemence of their objections to what he considered a perfectly ordinary and justifiable act. The India Office's mild put-down of the National Anthem spat as a non-issue not only failed to appreciate the threat Curzon saw to his constitutional superiority, but also (in assuming that the Governors would just need a light suggestion to stop playing the anthem) the Governors' cherishing of an act they saw as establishing the distinction between their presidencies and the rest of India, and their comparative equality to the Viceroy, as opposed to other Lieutenant Governors.

But the easy-going Hamilton was not cognisant of this underplay of psychological warfare, and it was not until repeated breaches of protocol and administrative lacunae in Madras were brought before him by Curzon that he ventured to pronounce that, 'Madras is detached because there is little going on in that sleepy presidency of sufficient importance to necessitate references to the India Office.'[52] The implication was there was not much lost due to Madras' un-communicativeness. Of course the same justification could be used to argue that the Governors of Madras should not be allowed the privilege of corresponding directly with the Secretary of State, as did the Viceroy, but Curzon did not employ it, preferring to base his arguments of theories of precedence and constitutional superiority.

It was not just Ampthill who was at fault though, but the entire character of the Madras cadre. Madras, according to Curzon, was 'out-of-the-way, and consumed with a sense of its own importance exactly proportionate to the consciousness that most people regard 'it as a somewhat insignificant and second class concern . . . pretensions [in Madras] have always been pushed more fiercely than in Bombay.'[53] Ampthill was eventually recognised and made acting Viceroy, perhaps at the instance of the India Office, where Godley held him in high esteem, once venturing to rebuke the Viceroy that he, Godley, would 'venture to say positively that Ampthill is *not* incompetent.'[54] Hamilton seems to have been less sanguine, attempting to console Curzon by stating his belief that Curzon would find 'that the social and ceremonial side of the Viceroyalty would be maintained at a very high level while you were away.'[55]

Contemporary scholars have also backed the contention that the administration of the Madras Presidency was not so very bad because, 'If association with the administration of Fort St. George immediately and of itself produced the force with which officials could smash the hegemonies of non-officials and establish their own rule'—a reference to the superimposition of an anglicised structure over local hierarchies of administration—'then that administration must have been very powerful and must have been able to command in society an overwhelming preponderance of force.'[56] Which it would not have been capable of doing if it were not efficient enough to hold the public trust.

The basic problem, then, lay with the system of governance that Curzon had to ensure that the Madras government functioned as a part of, and the channels through which he had to direct its administration. The system of Madras governance may have worked all right—at half-speed—when applied to Madras Presidency in isolation, but it would not do when faced with the exigencies of being tied to the Government of India, which in turn was tied to Whitehall and the larger currents of Empire. Madras had to be efficient in order to serve the interests of the Empire.[57] This was not the attitude of people in Madras; even though it was a 'very inferior outpost'[58] of Empire, the absence of local political institutions meant that the Governor of Madras could rule like an absolute ruler, and there was as much intrigue around him as around the Indian Princes, though this was by no means restricted to Madras alone; Curzon famously complained about Northcote being overshadowed by his two scheming Council Members.

The imperfection of Madras administration across all levels was noted even by its own Governor. In a breaking of ranks, Ampthill grumbled— but significantly, like his predecessor to George Hamilton and not the Viceroy—about the ease with which peasants could bribe revenue collectors to say that their crops were withered or destroyed, so that they could then claim exemption from paying land revenue.[59] Its other problem was the lack of a developmental vision and an unwillingness to break with bureaucratic tradition; in 1900, residents of Tirupati asked that the expenses for the local Girls' School, hitherto borne by the Municipality, be shouldered by the Madras Government, but Havelock refused, as it 'had no precedent.'[60]

But it is certainly true that despite their contretemps, the Curzon–Ampthill reign was effective in bringing British ideas of rule into Madras Presidency, in the spheres of Curzon's most cherished reforms. One of these was negating the effects of casteism. Ampthill actively prevented the formation of caste cliques by appointing one C. Sankara Nair as High Court Judge over one V. Krishnaswami Iyer because 'he (Sankara Nair) is not a Brahmin,'[61] and the previous three had been Brahmins. Of course, as Copland has noted elsewhere, the destruction of Brahmin preponderance in upper administrative positions was taken with British interests in mind as well.[62] This is illustrative of the streak of humanitarianism that runs through the administrations of both Curzon and Ampthill. Curzon stood up for the rights of Indians in cases like those of the 9th Lancers and for Indian labourers on Assam tea plantations; in Madras, in a similar instance on a Travancore plantation, Ampthill, backed by Curzon had the sentence condemning a planter who had killed an Indian confirmed. He also grumbled about the Foreign Department of the Government of India recommending that Indians get honours a degree lower than those recommended.[63] Ampthill proved himself in other areas as well. In spite of complaints from Curzon and the India Office about the slow pace of administration, even the political situation in Madras could be termed satisfactory. By 1904, the Congress and the Madras Mahajan Sabha were near collapse, because the local government stopped attending to their petitions, and therefore it began to be seen as 'not-respectable' i.e., affiliation to it probably did not advance one's prospects. Ampthill had the satisfaction of reporting to London the gratifying news that the 'Congress as it is worked at present is nothing more than an annual '*tamasha*' . . . a minor organization.'[64] Like Havelock, Ampthill also went in for more practical ways of elevating the status of Madras, such as fostering economic development. A note by one of his cadre suggests the holding of exhibitions and local museums showcasing each town's produce, such as Calcutta's then Economic Museum, a precursor to the Government Handicraft Emporiums of today.[65] It is thus apparent that the discovery of common ideals of administration improved Curzon's relations with Ampthill, and by extension, Simla–Madras relations as well.

AMPTHILL AS VICEROY

Ampthill, however, only became Acting Viceroy by default. It had largely been the availability of Northcote taking over as Acting Viceroy that had induced Curzon to suggest that he take leave in 1904 before embarking on his second term; he had himself suggested that the senior of the two Governors of Madras and Bombay fill this role; and at that time, Northcote (appointed just before Ampthill) had been the senior.[66] He was hugely disappointed when Northcote accepted an Australian appointment in 1903.[67] He was not too keen that Ampthill get the Viceregal spot, even though he respected Ampthill's administrative methods, partly because he thought the latter 'has a portentous sense of his own importance,' but mostly because 'you cannot take a man of thirty-four and make him head of the Government of India even for 4 or 5 months unless he is a very exceptional personality.'[68] Apparently, the Viceroy did think of his own self at least as a somewhat exceptional personality, as he had thought himself fit to take on the same office at thirty-nine. Curzon also had reservations about how Ampthill would be received by the senior bureaucrats in Simla; he predicted that Ampthill would be greeted with a 'good deal of suspicion and consternation . . . the high officials . . . do not know the higher sides of his intellect, his character, or his work, but everyone in India is aware of the fact that he is pompous and pedantic to a degree.'[69]

As a means of getting around this, he appointed J.O. Miller to be Ampthill's Private Secretary (Lawrence was retiring); apart from being an experienced, respected, and capable bureaucrat, Miller was also the son-in-law of Sir Alfred Lyall.

It would appear that Ampthill himself was aware of his position, writing to Lamington anxiously in May 1904 that he felt would 'have been more appropriate and generally satisfactory if the duty of acting as Viceroy had fallen to your lot, since you are my senior not only in years but also . . . in political and administrative experience.'[70]

But while he may have been suitably—and perhaps unnecessarily, as he did a good job—modest about his Viceregal capabilities, Ampthill certainly did not shrink from asserting the prerogatives of himself as Madras Governor. In his very first business letter to Lamington as Viceroy, he touched on what Curzon would have fumed at as the most provincial of subjects; the right of letting bands play the National Anthem for the Governors of Bombay and Madras. Since he had 'heard' that the loss of this 'ancient privilege' had caused Lamington as much vexation as it did him, he saw fit to mention, entirely between themselves, that if Lamington 'made a fight for the lost privilege' he, Ampthill, would stand by him. But of course, he hastily went on, he could 'hardly take advantage of my present position and raise the matter again.'[71]

In all fairness to Ampthill, he did his best to carry on the administration 'in faithful adherence of Lord Curzon's views and policy in matters both great and small,'[72] the matter in this case being to dissuade the Raj Saheb of Dhrangadra (or more usually spelt Dhrangadhra) from sending the Crown Prince to school in England. This could be indicative not only of Ampthill's sensible cognisance of his position, but also of Curzon's ability to inspire loyalty. (At this point, Ampthill was very strongly placed to become the next Viceroy, and striking an independent line could have brought him more notice.) It might also indicate that Ampthill as Governor of Madras was not being wilfully provoking, but merely responding to either needs of, or being infected by, the atmosphere at Madras; Curzon would have inclined to the latter.

There are many reasons as to why the Curzon–Ampthill relationship settled down to one of professional respect after the early days, the chief being a power vacuum in the immediate layer below the Viceroy and his Council, i.e., the Governors. In 1901, MacDonnell retired, and was followed in 1903 by Northcote, who went off to Australia. The previous year Sir John Woodburn of Bengal, whom Curzon greatly respected, had died suddenly. This left Ampthill as the senior-most and longest serving Governor, apart from Fryer of Burma (who also retired in 1903) in the country, and that too of a major administrative unit. By 1903, he would, in addition, have had considerable experience of working, and working in tandem with the Viceroy. He had never served under any other Viceroy and would thus be less likely to bring up counterpoints of administrative strategy. All this made him the ideal man to be Curzon's liaison point outside of the Viceroy's Council. In fact, by 1903, when both Northcote and Ampthill were in charge, there was a much vaunted amity between the Viceroy and the Governors generally; Northcote even insisted on seeing all the letters from all Departments of the Bombay Administration before they were sent off to the Viceroy.[73] He detailed to the Viceroy (thus breaking ranks with his subordinates) his uneasiness at grappling with the Bombay administration and judiciary over the Fernandez–Wray case.[74] This is indicative of the fact that he never tried to gloss over the troubles in his presidency and present a united front to the Government of India; but Ampthill's fighting spirit and willingness to stick up for his charges made him a better leader of men, and therefore more suited to the top spot than Northcote would have been.

However much Ampthill may have been obsessed with ceremonial, it could not be denied that he was devoted to his presidency. After stepping down as Acting Viceroy, he was offered, and refused, an Undersecretary-ship in London, because he felt that it was Madras which deserved to benefit from the 'unique experience and no amount of influence' he had accumulated as Viceroy. It would be unfair to deprive the Madras Presidency of those two factors in efficient administration. . . .'[75] Ampthill's staying on, unfortunately, did not much benefit either Madras or himself. He was pulled into the thick of intrigue over the Kitchener affair, which ensured that the Secretary of State did not devolve much time to the actual niceties of Indian administration,[76] and his vocal support of Curzon's stance cost him the Viceroyalty once Curzon resigned, as well as high office immediately after.

BOMBAY: 'INSUBORDINATION', TWICE OVER

Far from being a backwater, the other presidency, Bombay, was a bustling, mercantile presidency, largely devoted to commerce. It was not plagued by either ethnic or communal tensions, nor did it have any outstanding territorial realignment issues to be resolved. Nor was it ethnically divided, given that its two major groups, Gujaratis and Marathas, were largely split up between British India and princely India. As Curzon himself acknowledged in an address to the Bombay Municipality in 1900, 'one calamity which we have been fortunate enough to escape . . . is warfare in our own territory or upon our frontiers.'[77]

But unlike other presidencies and provinces, the Governor in Bombay was not top-dog. Bombay was an 'unwieldy Presidency',[78] with no one dominant power block. As far as British administrators went, Bombay throughout the late nineteenth century was a presidency dominated by the likes of Sir William Lee-Warner, whose specialism was in the Indian states. Apart from that, the city was dominated by its merchant chambers and industrial classes, whose concerns were commerce not politics, whatever Sir P.M. Mehta might say to the contrary.[79] To the hinterland of the Mahratta ghats the princelings of the old confederacy kept up a stir, and around Kathiawar, an entire block of the presidency was occupied by princely states, over which the Governors' writ did not directly run, and they were mostly much too small to be troublesome anyway. To some extent the situation was replicated in Madras, where the south Indian social structure took care of itself, in spite of Ampthill's *de-Brahminising* efforts. The opportunities for a Governor to make a splash were limited, and his duties covered varied specialisms, and given Bombay conditions during Curzon's time, the Viceroy was on the spot when he described the troubles of the Governor of Bombay as reminiscent of 'the afflictions of Job'.[80] Three successive governors— Sandhurst, Northcote and Lamington—tried and failed to make a constructive impact on a presidency ravaged by plague, famine, political insurrection, a nascent Congress movement and the depredations of its own Secretariat.

Sandhurst, the first, faced a presidency ravaged by plague, and the greater part of his term was spent in battling plague, famine and the Natu brothers. Curzon on arrival threw his support behind the Bombay governor, publicly praising him, especially commending his efforts at plague prevention and rehabilitation: 'The unceasing and devoted efforts of your rulers . . . in this place of your Governor, whose application to the onerous work . . . has excited widespread gratitude and admiration.'[81] He went on to describe Sandhurst as 'an untiring and chivalrous commander . . .'[82] in the fight against plague.

However, this was no more than the public closing of ranks among the governing elite. Curzon, popularly perceived as strongly anti-sedition, took an extremely balanced view of its so-called perpetrators within the Bombay Presidency. The Natu brothers, not convicted of shooting Rand and Ayerst in 1897, still languished in prison, and Curzon got to work to get the Bombay government to release them as fast as possible. This may have endeared him to the people, but not the Bombay officials who were responsible for persecuting the brothers in the first place, and might have left them feeling unsupported by the person who they had a right to believe should have backed them up. Sandhurst stalled; Curzon kept up the pressure. As a matter of fact the Curzon–Sandhurst correspondence shows a degree of harried acquiescence on Sandhurst's part as to the clearing of the two brothers; even then the release took nine months. The Natus were unconditionally released in December 1900, after Curzon had started pressuring the Government from March that year.

But as with the plague, Sandhurst, as well as his successor Northcote, displayed a spirit of exemplary cooperation and coordination with the centre when it came to famine relief. The centrally appointed Famine Relief Commission was headed by Sir A.P. MacDonnell, who had successfully tided Bengal and UP over famines in the past quarter-century. It is a testament to their overcoming their ingrained parochialism, and also to MacDonnell's administrative abilities, that there was no protest at his heading the Commission. It was, of course, a different matter when it was mooted that he might succeed as Governor of Bombay, as will be mentioned later in the chapter. MacDonnell's brusque style of functioning (detailed in the following chapter), and his quick decision-making abilities, as during the Cawmpore riots, might be Curzon's governing ideal, but it was far removed from that the Bombay governors happened to be. Curzon, apprehending protests from the Bombay cadre, ultimately gave way. MacDonnell left India in 1903. Sandhurst's successor was Lord Northcote, and not Alfred Lyall, who had also been mooted, but had declined citing a lack of enthusiasm.

Northcote was a greatly more efficient administrator than Sandhurst, yet the essential problems in the Bombay–Simla relationship remained the same. The Bombay Government and its Secretariat had a long history of open hostility to the Government of India, as they fought for control of the Princely States and overseas territories conquered under its aegis and with its army. Salisbury, Northbrook, and Lytton all complained about the fact that, at Secretariat level, the Bombay Government was 'imbued with a powerful and distinct sense of corporate identity, a compound of historical tradition and administrative pride.' Given this, the 'readiness of the local government to seek a confrontation with Calcutta was inspired as much by narrow feelings of parochialism and sectional rivalry as by a genuine desire to find a solution to the problem of divided control.'[83]

As noted above, this tendency was apparent in Madras too, but the problems faced by Curzon in relation to the 'insubordination' of Bombay and Madras were, while similar on the surface, of quite different character. While in both cases it was 'entirely wrong that the deliberate orders of the Home Government should be openly . . . ignored,' in Madras this took the form of 'knowing' ignorance, but in Bombay, perhaps because of the incompetence of the incumbent Governors during Curzon's time, government orders were 'likely quite unknowingly' ignored.[84] This was a dual irritant, all the more so because unlike Madras, a Viceroy, especially one who laid as much stress on foreign policy as Curzon, could not afford to forget about Bombay. Given that the territories they managed included princely states and some offshore colonies, Bombay—and its prickly political department—was in fact required to work very closely with the Viceroy, as well as the centrally appointed Famine Relief Commission, given the extent of famines across the presidency, from the princely states of Kathiawar to the border regions of Belgaum. In Curzon's time these problems, caused by the Bombay cadre's having a spirit of its own, were exacerbated by the fact that a series of weak Governors occupied office in succession. As Curzon and Hamilton realised, the system tended to overpower individual Governors brought in from the outside and unfamiliar with the administrative nuances of the 'most specialised service in the world.' Hamilton observed that the 'Civil Services, both of Madras and Bombay, are no doubt unduly sensitive as to interference, and in consequence much too secretive.'[85] He further attributed the intransigence of both Havelock and Northcote to the fact that,

> both no doubt have around them officials who wish to assert an independence that does not belong to the minor Presidencies, but that makes [their] position all the harder if [they] wish to cooperate with you, as the whole *entourage* become united in opposition to the legitimate authority and rights of the Indian Government.[86]

The extremely parochial nature of the Bombay cadre meant that the Governor also became something of a go-between and/or (but mostly and) scapegoat between them and the Government of India, as Northcote very aptly described to Curzon. Petitions from the Bombay cadre for increases in salaries and related matters could be sent up to the Viceroy at the Governor's discretion. Deluged under petitions (for the Bombay cadre was notoriously underpaid and unabashedly vocal about this injustice), Northcote refused to send up any but the strongest cases, and the resultant effect, as he wrote to Curzon, was 'a feeling that I, who have been fewer months in India than my colleagues have been years, in the face of their deliberate advice, refuse—not an increase of salary, but . . . the right to ask India if [AB] has not earned an increase of pay.'[87] This might also highlight the fact that the Bombay cadre did not see any hope of equitable treatment arising out of their sent-on petitions; certainly they seemed to see themselves as downtrodden compared to the other provinces. Their logic was that, 'India could hardly have refused [AB's request] when BC and DE in the Punjab and Madras have more pay and less work to do and so on.'[88] It is interesting that there are no direct hints of the Governor colluding with the Government of India (given that he was an external superimposition) to 'oppress' the Bombay cadre. This is also evidence that the various departments responsible for the running of India did not always pull together as a harmonious whole, and that 'regional and departmental loyalties hampered the coordination of Imperial policy.'[89]

Northcote could not escape the system; as noted, any incoming Governor was very quickly set upon by the two Councillors appointed to assist him, and Curzon gloomily admitted that even the fairly competent Northcote, whom he wished to stand in as Viceroy while he went to England on leave in 1904, was 'not strong enough to hold his own against his two Councillors, who are, of course, veteran partisans of the Bombay system.'[90] To illustrate to Hamilton how the system exerted its influence even over external Governors who should not have been imbued with provincial partisanship, Curzon cited the case of the Raja of Morvi, who, jealous of the fact that the Viceroy was going to visit the Rao of Cutch but not himself on his impending tour of Western India, asked for permission to sail to Europe three weeks before the Viceregal visit, pleading sickness. Northcote privately told the Viceroy he would not recommend granting of the request, but a week later made a formal recommendation in his capacity as Governor of Bombay that leave should be granted, indicative of the 'entire difference between the Governor when he meets the Viceroy or writes in independence of his Secretariat, and the Governor when he is once again under their influence.'[91] Curzon refused to grant leave in the event.

But it was also impossible to abolish the system of Executive Councils in Bombay and Madras, and thus water down the influence of the secretariat on what was supposed to be an impartial Governor, as long as English peers or politicians came out as Governors, as the incumbent would then need local advice, not having experienced those specific conditions of administration before.[92] This meant the members of the Governor's Council would continue to attempt to dominate the incumbent, whereas an ICS man with Indian experience would have been able to handle them effectively, though Curzon did not think so. As he observed to Lamington,

> So long as Governors are appointed from the outside they [Executive Councils] appear to me as great a necessity there, as a Council, for instance, is to the Viceroy here, and I would not dream of proposing their abolition. But in provinces headed by a Civilian, I would still less dream of introducing

a mechanism so fraught, under those conditions, with possibilities of friction and delay.[93]

And it was not considered desirable in Curzon's time to appoint an ICS man as a Governor in Bombay or Madras, because 'a great deal of the Congress Movement is based upon dislike and jealousy of the ICS, and if we give to them the monopoly of appointments in India, this feeling would be accentuated. It also has its reflections in Parliament . . .'[94] It would also have had a good deal to do with the belief of aristocratic competence, given that these Governors, already of noble birth, were usually further loaded with titles before they sailed out to take office.[95] So the situational deadlock stayed.

This scenario was the main reason why Curzon had so vainly pressed (and been refused) for Northcote's successor at Bombay someone who would not be overwhelmed by advice from his subordinates, because 'Government by one man is infinitely better than government by three men.'[96] He had asked for MacDonnell,[97] even though he had by then become disillusioned about what he had initially taken to be MacDonnell's lack of a desire for self-aggrandisement, over the issue of Victoria Memorial Funds, as he was the 'only efficient Indian Civilian' around. But nobody else wanted MacDonnell in Bombay because of his unpopularity with his officers and also the fact that he would be seen as an outsider by the Bombay cadre, making them even more obstructive. Finally, MacDonnell went back to London and a seat on the India Council, and Lord Lamington succeeded Northcote. Curzon acquiesced in the appointment of Lord Lamington only because there was no other option and since 'dependent upon me as he [Lamington, he was Best Man at Curzon's wedding] has always been, in India I am sure he will not lift a little finger without consulting me in advance.'[98] This would, of course, effectively bring the Bombay Presidency under the Government of India's thumb. Curzon's biographers have noted that he was the kind of leader who would prefer to work with a competent enemy rather than an unskilled well-wisher, but it is apparent that if the choice was between two unskilled persons, he would prefer to choose the one he considered himself to be capable of exercising more influence over, thus effectively steering the administration away from disaster.

Lamington was hardly unskilled. Curzon might console himself with the thought that the new Governor could be guided away from adminis- trative disaster given the Viceroy's influence over him, but as a matter of fact Lamington was eminently suited to the Bombay Governorship. It was his first posting since his term as governor of drought ridden Queensland from 1895–1901.[99] He seems to have hit the ground running, and within a fortnight of landing, had addressed issues regarding administration, police, Indian states (two cases), public expenditure, the Aga Khan, and pollution in Calcutta. And his old connections with the Viceroy did not prevent his making a stand for his presidency; when Curzon proposed that Aden be placed under Central command, Lamington admitted that it was 'difficult to justify its retention [by Bombay].' But, he went on, if Aden were to be 'removed from Bombay, then it should be considered whether Baroda should not be put again under Bombay. It is inextricably mixed up with the administration of Bombay.[100]

Thus, even while Curzon fulminated at the process which saw a 'titled ornamental' take the top spot in Bombay because it hampered the administration, it may well have been the optimum method of reducing friction between the Viceroy and the presidencies. A governor drafted in might be influenced by pressures from senior officials from that presidency's cadre (such as with Northcote and Sandhurst, and then again he might ultimately *not* be, such as what happened with Ampthill). Appointing a senior ICS person from a presidency to the top spot would invariably have resulted in a total breakdown in communications, especially given the extremely parochial nature of the Bombay cadre. And, as pointed out above, an ICS man from another province would not have been accepted by the local secretariat. But, it might also be argued to the contrary, that the bringing in of external people definitely contributed to a lack of political continuity at Bombay; an ICS man would not have had the same incentive as Northcote, for instance, did, to accept other, possibly more prestigious appointments mid-way through his term.[101]

It was not just a case of persons alone, though the Home Government seems to have construed it as such. Nor can it be said that all the Governors were wilful insubordinates, or that Curzon tarred them all with the same brush, because of which they and their presidencies became more uncooperative than ever. Letters from Hamilton and Godley solely cogitate as to the most suitable (or least unsuitable) person who could be appointed as Sandhurst's successor to the Bombay Governorship, as though a change of persona at the top would solve all problems, especially if that individual and the incumbent Viceroy were in agreement over the issues at stake. But, as Curzon was to argue, and as happened with the successor eventually chosen, the system proved more overpowering than the individual.[102] It was the system Curzon complained about, a system that needed a strong person to override it, and also to effect the changes the Viceroy wanted. The influence of a particular presidency's work culture upon a newly drafted Governor was telling across most presidencies, but it was in Bombay that it was at its height. At Madras, even though Havelock left detailed notes for his successor as to the Simla–Madras relationship,[103] seemingly designed to sabotage any hope of a smooth working relationship with Curzon and the said successor, Ampthill eventually forged an efficient working style of his own, completing obliterating the bad blood that had existed between the Centre and Madras in Havelock's time. While Madras' isolation has often been cited as a reason for its keeping aloof from Government of India proceedings, and the potential for sulking over (imaginary?) slights passed at their rare meetings and interactions, Bombay's very close relationship to the centre demanded extensive contact, multiplying the possibilities for friction, especially on shared subjects. One must also take into account the situations or governing climates which diverse governors were called upon to face, not only with regard to the exigencies of exceptional crises like famines, but day-to-day administration as well. As Curzon said, 'A street crowd in Lahore does not present the smallest resemblance to one in Bombay. Bombay is utterly unlike Calcutta.'[104] For example, the Bombay Presidency was never very political, i.e., not rife with issues of ethnic and communal tensions. The concerns facing the Bombay Secretariat were, on the one hand, their semi-autonomous foreign policy—and this was greatly reduced following the removal of their off-shore dependencies and major princely states like Baroda to the command of the Government of India. By Curzon's time, therefore, the concerns of the Bombay Government were primarily those of 'repressing sedition'. Madras was not as politically turbulent, and once the chief causes of friction, i.e., administrative inefficiency and A.E. Havelock—were removed, it became something of a model presidency. Therefore, it was a combination of the temper of the presidency and the personality of the Governor, as well as specific situational contexts that determined Bombay and Madras' reactions to Curzon and his reforms.

INTER-PRESIDENCY RIVALRY

In part the cribbing of the Governors, and their jockeying for status and precedence, stemmed from inter-provincial rivalry. Inter-presidency equations were dominated by rival claims to being the most privileged, and autonomous, presidency. Even the ordering of precedence found its way into inter-presidential rivalries. An Indian prince might refuse to attend the Durbar because he felt he was being slighted by not being granted precedence over any of his contemporaries; but this was very much the concern of the Governors of the Presidencies too. Precedence was set by dualistic, and sometimes duelling, factors. This could, and did, cause confusion at the Delhi Durbar. Between Bombay and Madras, the 'precedence of Madras over Bombay [was] an immutable historical and official fact,' but in the Warrant of Precedence, 'within a particular group precedence [was] decided by the date at which the individuals within the group entered it.'[105] The upshot of this sociological sounding epithet was that Northcote would take precedence over Ampthill at Delhi as he had come out to India as Governor of Bombay slightly

before Ampthill came out to take charge of Madras. At the Durbar
Ampthill considered that the Governors had been slighted, and asked
Northcote to collaborate in drawing up a list of slights apparently
suffered by the two Governors, in an attempt at provincial solidarity.
Northcote declined, and Curzon, writing to Hamilton, described him
as the 'most sensible and loyal little man in the world,'[106] a patronising
label that nonetheless reflected the stolid qualities preferable in a
Governor if a mercurial leader like MacDonnell was not on hand. On
the other hand, we have seen how Ampthill worked to establish cordial
relations with the Governor of Bombay when he was appointed Viceroy
over Lamington. Thus, there was certainly inter-presidential jealousy
over precedence and status with Simla, but there was no real hatred/
rivalry, this being reserved for Simla and the provinces closer to it, which
were seen as hogging more than their fair share of benefits from the
Centre.

In conclusion, it may be said that there was no genuine animosity
between Curzon and the Governors of the major Presidencies, nor did
they fall out over the handling of many political issues. While Curzon's
relations with Bombay and Madras were marked with an unvarying
degree of sameness, there was a unique aspect to his individual
interactions not only with the two Presidencies, but also with the
different incumbent Governors. Since the Governor was the figurehead
of these administrations, it was his relations with Curzon that could be
said to symbolize the Viceroy's relationship with the Presidency as a
whole. Thus we have the Governor acting as front man for his
administrations. At times, however, most notably in the case of Ampthill,
the Governor's relationship differed from, and changed, for the brief
period he was in office, the tempo of the Centre's equation with the
given province. Curzon had time to develop a personal equation with
Ampthill in Madras, but not so with Bombay because of the comparative
frequency with which Governors kept changing, so it is possible he saw
it and its administration in more generalized terms and did not engage
with it to the same degree of closeness with which he worked alongside

Ampthill to negotiate reforms. Also, Bombay's administration was on a war and not day-to-day footing for much of the time during Curzon's Viceroyalty, due to successive waves of plague, famine, and political unrest.

But it was not until the turbulent closing years of Curzon's Viceroyalty that the Presidency Governors, in the face of what they (along with Curzon) perceived as a conspiracy between the Indian Army and the Home Government, backed the Viceroy magnificently, in the process (at least in Ampthill's case), alienating themselves from London and political advancement. Until then, Havelock and Ampthill's using their privileges to write to the Secretary of State about being miffed at apparently cavalier treatment from Simla was cause enough to suspect that Curzon was right in wanting to remove this privilege. By 1905, it became apparent that it was the Home Government that was using this privilege to unsettle the Viceroy, and not the Presidency Governors. For instance, Ampthill once wrote a detailed letter to Brodrick about the day-to-day work of a Madras Governor, to which Brodrick replied that he did not have much to say on Madras questions before passing on to the latest Kitchener–Curzon gossip.[107] Ampthill very categorically recorded his distaste of the attempt by Balfour to use him as a source of information;[108] evidence that the apolitical thesis of administration in India had been imbibed by even an external, non-ICS Governor.

Nor do the Governors themselves, especially Ampthill, given his enhanced opportunities to get close to the centre of power, and the India Office's attempt to sedulously cultivate him as a counterpoise to Curzon, seem to have taken advantage of the frosty relationship between Curzon and the Balfour–Brodrick duo; evidence of the fact that if decentralization as envisaged by the British Cabinet was meant to function as a means of crosschecking Viceregal power, it was a failure. It may have been because the Governors were not politically influential or politically inclined men back home; in any case, official relationships between the Governors and the India Office do not seem to have been deep-rooted or personal, but rather, mainly confined to a bit of official cribbing so

long as the protagonists were in office. By refusing to take part in that
most unsavoury of political intrigues, the Kitchener affair, the Presidency
Governors did show themselves to be administrators after the Curzon
ethos in the most critical spheres, the ethics of running an Empire.

Thus far, I have focussed on the relations of Curzon as a lone office
holder with his Governors. As Ampthill, and indeed Curzon himself
noted, in India the individual was paramount: 'In India . . . public
opinion . . . attributes every act of Government to the individual will
and personality of its head.'[109] But there was more to the Government
of India. Outside of Madras and Bombay the presence of the ICS was
more strongly felt, and the Governor was always an ICS man. It was the
province of Punjab, and its incumbent Governor, that Curzon engaged
with much more combatively than he was ever compelled to with
Bombay and Madras put together. This chapter has illustrated how
individual relations shaped perceptions of Curzon's government in
London. The next chapter explores how Curzon engaged with the less
political, but more bureaucratic heads of the provinces of British India.

Notes

1. Ampthill to Curzon, 05 September 1905, Curzon Papers, Mss Eur F111/211.
2. Amit Kumar Gupta, *Between a Tory and a Liberal: Bombay under Sir James Fergusson, 1880–1885*, (Calcutta: K.P. Bagchi and Co., 1978), p. 5.
3. William Rose Mansfield, 1st Viscount Sandhurst, GCSI, GCIE, GCVO, PC (1855–1921), Governor of Bombay (1895–1900).
4. Henry Stafford Northcote, 1st Baron Northcote GCMG, GCIE, CB, PC (1846–1911), Governor of Bombay, (1900–1903).
5. Charles Wallace Alexander Napier Ross Cochrane-Baillie, 2nd Baron Lamington (1860–1940), Governor of Bombay (1903–1907).
6. Arthur Oliver Villiers Russell, 2nd Baron Ampthill (1869–1935), Governor of Madras (1900–1906) and Acting Viceroy (1904).
7. Curzon to Havelock, 11 September 1899, Curzon Papers, Mss Eur F111/200.
8. *Le Maistre*, 'The Second Baron Ampthill's Governorship of Madras and Viceroyalty', X.
9. Curzon to Havelock, 11 September 1899, Curzon Papers, Mss Eur F111/200.
10. Ampthill to Lamington, 21 May 1904, Lamington Papers. Mss Eur B159.

11. John Martineau, *The Life and Correspondence of Sir Bartle Frere, Vol. 1*, (London: John Murray, 1895), p. 418.

12. Martineau, *Life of Sir Bartle Frere, Vol.1*, p. 418.

13. Table XIII, *Gazetteer of the Bombay Presidency, Surat-Broach, Vol. II–B*, (Bombay: Printed at the Government Central Press, 1904), p. 13.

14. Ampthill to Hamilton, 26 June 1901, Ampthill Papers, Mss Eur E233/9.

15. Curzon to Havelock, 11 September 1899, Curzon Papers, Mss Eur F111/200.

16. The point here is not whether the force was needed or not, or whether Havelock's request was justified. The narrative is meant to illustrate the uses and services and contested expressions of power.

17. Ampthill to Curzon, 27 February 1902, Curzon Papers, Mss Eur F111/205.

18. Sir Arthur Elibank Havelock (1844–1908), Governor of Madras 1896–1900.

19. Havelock to Curzon, 18 August 1899, Havelock Papers, Mss Eur D699.

20. See Chapter 3, p. 123.

21. Curzon to Hamilton, 17 May 1899, Curzon Papers, Mss Eur F111/158.

22. Curzon to Hamilton, 31 May 1899, Curzon Papers, Mss Eur F111/158.

23. Curzon to Godley, 12 July 1899, Curzon Papers, Mss Eur F111/158.

24. R.J. Moore, Foreword, in Gupta, *Between a Tory and a Liberal*.

25. Ampthill to Brodrick, 14 and 16 June 1905, Ampthill Papers, Mss Eur E233/7/2; and Brodrick to Ampthill, 7 July 1905, Ampthill Papers, Mss Eur E233/12.

26. The Bombay Presidency: Report of a Speech given by Sir William Lee-Warner, at the Society of the Arts, 15 January 1904. Press cutting in the Richardson Collection, Mss Eur C276.

27. Rt. Hon. Lord George Hamilton, *Parliamentary Reminiscences and Reflections 1886–1906*, (London: John Murray, 1922), p. 298.

28. This section about the NWFP is meant to illustrate how interventionist policies were needed when the Punjab administration was found to be lacking; the same imperatives did not apply to Madras. Also this, in a way, mirrors the taking away of Aden and Baroda from Bombay command earlier, which does not fall into the time frame covered by this thesis.

29. Curzon to Hamilton, 31 May 1899, Curzon Papers, Mss Eur F111/158.

30. Memorandum by the Viceroy on the NWFP (Wording), Curzon Papers, Mss Eur F111/322, pp. 12–13.

31. Curzon to Hamilton, 29 August 1900, Curzon Papers, Mss Eur F111/159.

32. More than Mackworth Young himself, it was his wife who carried on the anti-Curzon campaign on the terraces of Simla after Mackworth Young took offence at the way the NWFP affair was handled, at one instance cutting the Viceroy at church.

33. Lamington to Curzon, 13 October 1904, Lamington Papers, Micro reel 675, 26–7, in Copland, 'The Bombay Political Service, 1863–1924', p. 295.

34. Havelock to Curzon, 19 June 1899, Havelock Papers, Mss Eur D699/2 (Letter Book 2).

35. Havelock to Curzon, 11 July 1899, Havelock Papers, Mss Eur D699/2.

36. One of the bitterest letters of the Curzon–Havelock correspondence occurred when Havelock, on tour, inaugurated a bridge, subsequently called the Havelock Bridge, that the Viceroy was to have declared open.

37. Curzon to Hamilton, 23 February 1899, Curzon Papers, Mss Eur F111/158.

38. Curzon to Hamilton, 02 March 1899, Curzon Papers, Mss Eur F111/158.

39. Curzon to Hamilton, 20 September 1899, Curzon Papers, Mss Eur F111/158.

40. Extract of letter from Havelock to Hamilton, 24 May 1899, enc. in letter, Hamilton to Curzon, 16 June 1899, Curzon Papers, Mss Eur F111/158.

41. Havelock to Curzon, 11 July 1899, Havelock Papers, Mss Eur D699/2.

42. Havelock to Curzon, 18 August 1899, Curzon Papers, Mss Eur F111/200.

43. Hamilton to Curzon, 05 September 1900, Hamilton Papers, Mss Eur C126/2.

44. ATP, 'Powers and Prerogatives appertaining under Statute by Ordinance or by usage, to the Governors of Madras and Bombay and to their Executive Councils as compared to those similarly appertaining to Lieutenant Governors and other heads of non-presidential Governments and Administrations, by ATP, 7 December 1900,' in Le Maistre, 'The Second Baron Ampthill's Governorship of Madras and Viceroyalty', Mss Eur D878, p. 215.

45. Curzon to Ampthill, 1 February 1901, Ampthill Papers Mss Eur 233/15.

46. Curzon to Hamilton, 22 January 1903, Curzon Papers, Mss Eur F111/162.

47. Curzon to Hamilton, 05 February 1903, Curzon Papers, Mss Eur F111/162.

48. Curzon to Hamilton, 05 February 1903, Curzon Papers, Mss Eur F111/162.

49. Hamilton to Curzon, 27 February 1903, Curzon Papers, Mss Eur F111/162.

50. Brodrick to Curzon, 20 January 1905, Midleton Papers, Add. Mss 50077.

51. Curzon to Brodrick, 02 February 1905, Midleton Papers, Add. Mss 50077.

52. Hamilton to Curzon, 08 June 1899, Curzon Papers, Mss Eur F111/158.

53. Curzon to Hamilton, 05 March 1903, Curzon Papers, Mss Eur F111/158.

54. Godley to Curzon, 14 August 1903, Curzon Papers, Mss Eur F111/158.

55. Hamilton to Curzon, 14 August 1903, Curzon Papers, Mss Eur F111/158.

56. Washbrook, The Emergence of Provincial Politics, p. 41.

57. Ibid., pp. 50–1.

58. Ibid., pp. 215–16.

59. Ampthill to Hamilton, 6 August 1902, Ampthill Papers, Mss Eur E233/5.

60. 'Address from, and Reply to, the People of Tirupati, in Addresses Presented to and Replies Delivered by H.E. Sir A.E. Havelock, GCMG GCIE, on his 15th Tour in the Madras Presidency, 1900', (Madras: Superintendent, Government Press, 1900), p. 984.

61. Ampthill to Hamilton, 8 September 1903, Ampthill Papers, Mss Eur E233, in Washbrook, Emergence of Provincial Politics, p. 283–4.

62. Ian Copland, *The British Raj and the Indian Princes*, p. 63.

63. *Le Maistre*, 'The Second Baron Ampthill's Governorship of Madras and Viceroyalty', p. 75.

64. Ampthill to Brodrick, 7 January 1904, Ampthill Papers, in Washbrook, *Emergence of Provincial Politics*, p. 231.

65. F.A. Nicholson, *Memo: Economic Development of India: Developing the Trade of India with Other Countries*, 23 November 1901, Ampthill Papers, Mss Eur E233/26. Sent to Campbell, Military Secretary to Ampthill.

66. Curzon to Balfour, 05 February 1903, Balfour Papers, Add. Mss 49732.

67. Northcote became only the second Governor General of Australia.

68. Curzon to Hamilton, 22 July 1903, Curzon Papers, Mss Eur F111/162.

69. Curzon to Brodrick, 28 October 1903, Midleton Papers, Add. Mss 50074.

70. Ampthill to Lamington, 1 May 1904, Lamington Papers, Mss Eur B159/1.

71. Ampthill to Lamington, 21 May 1904, Lamington Papers, Mss Eur B159/1.

72. Ampthill to Lamington, 21 May 1904, Lamington Papers, Mss Eur B159.

73. Northcote to Curzon, 30 April 1903, Curzon Papers, Mss Eur F111/207.

74. Northcote to Curzon, 04 March 1903, Curzon Papers, Mss Eur F111/207.

75. Ampthill to his mother, the Dowager Lady Russell, 12 January 1905, Russell Family Private Collection, in *Le Maistre*, 'The Second Baron Ampthill's Governorship of Madras and Viceroyalty', p. xii.

76. See Chapter 3, p. 138.

77. George Curzon, 'Reply to an Address from the Bombay Municipality', 8 November 1900, in *Lord Curzon in India: Being a Selection from his Speeches as Viceroy and Governor-General of India*, Sir Thomas Releigh (ed.), p. 25.

78. A.H.L. Fraser (President, Indian Police Commission) to Curzon, 15 December 1902, Curzon Papers, Mss Eur F111/206.

79. Sir P.M. Mehta, Speech at the Bombay Session of the INC, in *Notable Utterances at the National Congress of December 1904*, (n.p., n.d.).

80. Curzon to Sandhurst, 25 August 1899, Curzon Papers, Mss Eur F111/200.

81. George Curzon, 'Reply to address from the Bombay Municipality', 30 December 1898, in *Lord Curzon in India*, Sir Thomas Raleigh (ed.), p. 16.

82. George Curzon, Speech at Meeting of Voluntary Plague Workers, Poona, 11 November 1899, in ibid., p. 509.

83. Copland, 'The Bombay Political Service, 1863–1924', pp. 298–9.

84. Curzon to Hamilton, 8 April 1903, Curzon Papers, Mss Eur F111/162.

85. Hamilton to Curzon, confidential, undated, around end September 1900, Curzon Papers, Mss Eur F111/159. It is unclear as to why Hamilton refers to Bombay and Madras as 'minor', when clearly they were not.

86. Hamilton to Curzon, undated, private, August 1900, Curzon Papers, Mss Eur F111/159.

87. Northcote to Curzon, 26 February 1902, Curzon Papers, Mss Eur F111/205.

88. Northcote to Curzon, 26 February 1902, Curzon Papers, Mss Eur F111/205.

89. Copland, 'The Bombay Political Service, 1863–1924', p. 9.

90. Curzon to Hamilton, 20 June 1900, Curzon Papers, Mss Eur F111/159.

91. Curzon to Hamilton, 03 October 1900, Curzon Papers, Mss Eur F111/159.

92. Curzon to Brodrick, 05 April 1904, Curzon Papers, Mss Eur F111/163.

93. Curzon to Lamington, 27 February 1904, Curzon Papers, Mss Eur F111/209.

94. Hamilton to Curzon, 16 June 1899, Curzon Papers, Mss Eur F111/158.

95. David Cannadine, *Ornamentalism: How the British Saw Their Empire*, (London: Allen Lane/The Penguin Press, 2001), pp. 94–5.

96. Curzon to Brodrick, 28 January 1904, Curzon Papers, Mss Eur F111/163.

97. Curzon to Hamilton, 22 July 1903, Curzon Papers, Mss Eur F111/162.

98. Curzon to Hamilton, 19 August 1903, Curzon Papers, Mss Eur F111/162.

99. This fact is not likely to have endeared him to Curzon. While campaigning against the practice of outside appointments to Bombay and Madras in 1899, he had grumbled to Hamilton that it often resulted in a governor being transferred to India from the Crown Colonies, 'where he was a petty king, and who . . . transplant[s] to Indian soil the theories of his former station.' Curzon to Hamilton, 28 June 1899, Curzon Papers, Mss Eur F111/158. Cf. Curzon's line of thought with Mark Francis' assertion that by the late nineteenth century, governors of settler colonies started declaiming personal authority and representing themselves as 'symbolic representatives of the British monarch.' Francis, *Governors and Settlers,* p. 8. As Francis himself contends, this shift was brought about by pressures from England; it may therefore be conjectured that Curzon's ideas about the properly subordinate place his governors should occupy stemmed from his past as a Home politician and parliamentarian.

100. Lamington to Curzon, 16 April 1904, Curzon Papers, Mss Eur F111/209.

101. It is true that many ICS people did serve in other parts of the Empire, but not, however, in Governor General capacity, this being reserved for peers etc.

102. See above, p. 114.

103. See, for example, ATP, 'Powers and Prerogatives Appertaining under Statute by Ordinance or by Usage, to the Governors of Madras and Bombay', in *Le Maistre*, 'The Second Baron Ampthill's Governorship of Madras and Viceroyalty', Mss Eur D878, p. 215.

104. George Curzon, 'Reply to Address from the Bombay Municipality', 8 November 1900, in *Lord Curzon in India*, Sir Thomas Raleigh (ed.), p. 29.

105. Curzon to Northcote, 27 September 1902, Curzon Papers, Mss Eur F111/206.

106. Curzon to Hamilton, 13 January 1903, Curzon Papers, Mss Eur F111/162.

107. Brodrick to Ampthill, 07 July 1905, in *Le Maistre*, 'The Second Baron Ampthill's Governorship of Madras and Viceroyalty', p. 163.

108. Ampthill to his Mother, 07 August 1905, Russell Family Private Collection, in Le Maistre, 'The Second Baron Ampthill's Governorship of Madras and Viceroyalty',

165. Cf. Chapter 5. The same material has been used, albeit in a different context, to illustrate how the India Office attempted to utilise assumed friction between the Governors and Simla to their own advantage.

109. Ampthill to Brodrick, 12 May 1904, Ampthill Papers, Mss Eur E233/37.

4

The Provinces: The ICS and Its Head?

You have thought fit to treat me with marked discourtesy on a charge the evidence for which you will not disclose. . . . I am unable to accept with any satisfaction Your Excellency's appreciation

Sir Mackworth Young to Curzon,
February 1902

Much of the portraiture of Curzon in India that comes down to us is from the pens of the ICS (Indian Civil Service), some of whom were even better as historians than as administrators. It is the 'competition-*wallah's*' pen that has written the accepted caricature of Curzon: well-meaning, expert, over-enthusiastic and very caustic; it is in fact the one consensual agreement reached by modern historians and the 'Orientalists' they affect to critique. Philip Mason, Penderel Moon, Walter Lawrence and Harcourt Butler all essentially offer up the same unvarying analysis. There are chapters on Curzon in most major works about British India, the most extensive, informative and didactic is Penderel Moon's, *The British Conquest and Dominion of India*.[1] Moon's account is that of a civil servant of long-standing, its author taking for granted his right to interpret and judge a fellow administrator's actions. Appearing to co-opt 'efficiency of administration' Moon lists most of Curzon's domestic legislation as being constructive, his foreign policy rather less so, possibly because it was here that Curzon let his 'unwarranted' Russophobia intrude. But at the time, the threat from Russia was real, and it must be remembered that Russia did invade Afghanistan in 1979, and the spill-over has destabilised what is now Pakistan. By Moon's time, i.e., post the Great War, the Russian threat had receded, and Moon's view of Curzon is probably influenced by the greater importance of keeping internal order in his own time. Michael Edwardes' observation about the ultimate futility of Curzon's strenuous Viceregal undertakings[2] is echoed by Philip Mason in, *The Men Who Ruled India*,[3] for the same reason; Indians had by then begun to assert their own views for their future in a world indisposed to endorse the idea of a people being subject to another. This is, of course, more a reflection on the evolving attitudes of the ICS than their attitudes towards and assessment of the Viceroy.

If Curzon's relationship with the Governors of the presidencies offers an analysis of how he engaged with people he often did not think deserved to be in power, because of their lack of relevant expertise, then the provinces throw up clues as to how he could engage with a specialized bureaucracy whose top members could arguably said to be as knowledgeable, and perhaps more experienced, than him. What emerged at times was a struggle for power; each counterparty believing that his particular brand of knowledge was more suitable for the contemporary situation. Yet the ICS also offers a perfect model for examining the necessarily unequal power balance between Curzon and his subordinates, and how this was negotiated and worked around, given that Curzon, unlike Milner, has a reputation of not being subordinate-friendly, a reputation largely built upon the accounts of his subordinates. The relationship between the self-styled (albeit so that he could identify with its admired ethos) 'head of the ICS' and the rank and file was necessarily that between a chief and his subordinates; the Viceroy in India was *primus* and above, again due to a consciously adhered to warrant of precedence. An outstanding work in this context is Khalid bin Sayeed's, *Pakistan: The Formative Phase*,[4] a section of which explores the exact position of the Viceroy of India; was he the 'titular head of the Indian Civil Service,'[5] or the representative of the British Cabinet in India? While Sayeed answers this question with relevance to the Pakistan Movement, an analysis as to whether Curzon was of the governors or the administrators is pertinent because, by locating, or placing him within a certain ideological camp, we have a basis upon which to interpret his relations with both 'factions'. As discussed above, Curzon, with his 'middle-class method' and a Viceroyalty funded via an American merchandising empire, was avowedly not an *aristocratic* aristocrat, and yet this was invariably the position he occupied vis-à-vis the ICS. This chapter is thus also pertinent in analysing how the social backgrounds of the administrators of the Raj informed their constructions of politics and polity—a subaltern studies project whose subject is anything but subaltern.

During Curzon's term in India, many prominent civil servants were doing their spell of duty: Vincent Smith Commissioner of NWP and Oudh, 1898–1900; H.H. Risley, 1902–1905, Home Secretary to Government of India; Robert Nathan, Private Secretary to Curzon 1904–1905; John Ontario Miller, Private Secretary to Ampthill, 1904; Sir John Woodburn, Lieutenant Governor of Bengal 1898–1902; Sir William Mackworth Young, Lieutenant Governor of the Punjab 1897–1902; Sir T.W. Holderness, Secretary to Government of India for Revenue and Agriculture 1898–1901; Sir Antony Patrick MacDonnell, Lieutenant Governor of the United Provinces 1898–1901.[6] How did Curzon interact with, and impose his authority upon these senior administrators? What did ICS people think a Viceroy should be like? Did Curzon, according to them, go beyond his brief and intrude into their brief by being too enthusiastic about efficiency of administration? Did they feel disenfranchised or gratified? Just how was he perceived by the ICS and how did he engage with the Viceroy's Council? As with the Presidency Governors, the forming of mutual impressions and the recording of these for posterity was a two-way process between Curzon and the ICS. But being rather more his subordinates, the ICS men were not open to seeing Curzon's vulnerabilities, nor to watching his work at close quarters or through direct interaction. One must also take into account how the issues over which Curzon's relations with the senior ICS were structured influence the whole interpersonal relationships paradigm. For instance, Mackworth Young is generally held to have been the one at fault in his spat with Curzon; but had the governor of any other province been in the identical position of having a huge chunk of his territory lopped off and refashioned into a whole new province without being consulted, he too might have reacted in the same way. What, then, were the varied motives behind the diverse reactions and feedback Curzon sparked among the ICS?

Historians have not, however, made any in-depth analyses of Curzon's relationship with the ICS. Even Curzon's at time critical views about the ICS have not always been utilised by historians who seek to show that the ICS was not the machine of all encompassing efficiency that the memoirs of its old hands would have liked people to believe; they have just been used to illustrate Curzon's man-management skills—or lack of them. Those historians who take a high politics approach to the Curzon Viceroyalty tend to base their sources among the papers of eminent Conservative politicians, and confine the politics of power discussion to these circles. For those taking a more specifically Indian look at Curzon in India, such as Penderel Moon, the temptation is to dismiss him as having 'come from above', an alien if expert superimposition upon the most specialized service in the world. The traditional incompatibility of the ICS and the 'colonial governors'—differences due in part to class— has prevented synthesised studies of the two, except as opposing elements. Even more so, despite stressing the special administrative systems in place for Madras and Bombay, there are no parallel generalizations about how coming from the ICS affected Governors' relations with their Governor General. This chapter seeks to redress this gap in historiography using as case studies two Governors who had diametrically opposing relationships with Curzon. Curzon's highly approving assessment of Sir Antony MacDonnell, the UP Lieutenant Governor, has been used to illustrate the parameters under which Curzon could be said to have forged an ideal working relationship with a highly placed subordinate, and his often neglectful attitude towards Mackworth Young of the Punjab illustrates why so very many of his subordinates found him unduly harsh. As a binding theme, this chapter also examines Curzon's relations with the ICS, in terms of the power he exercised over them. It is built on two tiers, or levels of contact, the ICS had with the Viceroy as members of the Viceroy's Council and as senior administrators, along with the hypothesis that the latter had more active say in administrative affairs as they could be considered to be up-to-date on current affairs. The Viceroy's Council itself is examined in terms of its position in the Simla–Whitehall tussle for power that erupted after 1902.

Curzon's alleged dominance over the ICS is not a foregone conclusion; it must be remembered that while Curzon obviously had the upper hand—he *was* the Viceroy, and an acknowledged expert on eastern affairs, the ICS was a highly specialized body of men who had spent their lives mastering a particular subject in the field, and traditionally, as Judith Brown observes, the Viceroy of India had been (mostly always) an aristocrat with little previous knowledge of India, and had depended heavily upon his Home Department for advice.[7] Given this historical context, Curzon *could not* have come straight out and superimposed his views upon the ICS; indeed, it has been widely suggested he did not evoke strong reactions from the ICS, only a bemused scurrying around to carry out his plans, and peevish protestations when these were resented. He has done much to foster this impression himself, and in part because the administrators he approved of were people of long-standing approaching the end of their careers, there has not been much study of his long-term legacy on the men who ruled India. The one junior civilian who went on to attain prominence was Harcourt Butler, and his formative influence, it is widely assumed, was the setting of Oudh.

Offsetting the accounts produced by Mason and Moon, there is a purposefully short section about Curzon in India in Walter Lawrence's *The India We Served*, a first-hand account (and much quoted) by Curzon's private secretary of five years. Most of it stresses Curzon's prodigious capacity for unceasing work; and Lawrence also makes the interesting, and I believe, much unappreciated point that there were no communal clashes during Curzon's time in India, proof, according to

Lawrence, that Curzon's 'patient endeavour to hold the balance was not in vain.'[8] It is a discussion of Curzon's style of working more than an introspective piece into the details of his administration. Seen in contiguity with his account of pre-Curzonian India, Lawrence's work makes it possible to comprehend the statements of later writers as to why the ICS saw Curzon as a superimposition trying to exceed his brief. Lawrence's oft-quoted account recounts how many civil servants were extremely blasé about Curzon's appointment and cynical about his ability to effect changes; even among the senior bureaucrats, Curzon's appointment typically appears to have engendered bemusement, in part because he was an unknown quantity. Evan Maconochie recounts how his father-in-law, a senior civil servant, reacted to the news:

> Mr Ibbetson had given his life to India, had taken little leave, and was not in close touch with English politics and personalities. I remember him wondering at the time of Lord Curzon's appointment, 'what all the fuss was about.' He was soon to learn. From the time of association a bond of sympathy was established between the two which ripened into a warm mutual regard and admiration . . .[9]

Of course, biographers are quick to point out that Ibbetson's and A.P. MacDonnell's were isolated cases; predominantly, Curzon and the ICS failed to establish an easy working relationship. This included a good many of the governors. And this is crucial to assessing Curzon's working relationships and the nature of the bonds he established with his officers in India, because, in a very real sense, the ICS was the administration of India. It permeated everything. The members of the Viceroy's Council were primarily drawn from the senior ranks of the ICS, the India Council was—according to Curzon in his more irascible moods—a place for the ICS to throw a wet blanket over any Viceroy tampering with an administrative system they regarded as theirs, and of course, the Lieutenant Governorships of the provinces and Bengal. While the spotlight is often on the fact that the Viceroyalty (in practice) and the Governorships of Bombay and Madras were denied the heaven born— the fact is that the ICS controlled the most part of the administrative apparatus of the Indian Empire. In addition to the heads of all provinces except Bombay and Madras and the residents of the Princely States, Curzon's private secretaries—Walter Lawrence, J.O. Miller and Robert Nathan, and most members of his Viceroy's Council, were drawn from the ICS. And they had the ear of the India Office as well. Curzon's interaction with the ICS must not, therefore, be assessed within the narrow confines of the active servicemen he considered the Viceroy to be head of. What Curzon thought of the state of the ICS would have determined his approach to them, and this in turn set the pace for much of Centre-Provincial relations throughout Curzon's Viceroyalty and heavily influenced Curzon's approach to governance.

Kipling might write that an 'erring' ICS Assistant Commissioner would be told that he must remember that 'the service was made for the country and not the country for the service,' but this jesting satire carries the implication of a certainty that Kipling did not think that the ICS actually thought India was made for them. Fifteen years later, the man who is equated with Kipling as the arch proponent of Empire could write as though he actually feared that this was indeed the case; in a gloomy jeremiad, Curzon wrote to his temperate Secretary of State that,

> I cannot help feeling the truth of the contention that just now India is exploited for the benefit of the civil service, and that the statutory rights which they have obtained from long possession of a monopoly of government in India, and the increasing difficulty of in anyway ousting them from their position, or of stirring them up to the activity and the interest in the governed shown by their predecessors, is an increasing danger.[10]

This is significant not just because it expresses concern about the purported declining standards of a service touted as the backbone of British administration in India, but because, as theorised above, such a view would have had a direct impact on Curzon's attitude to that service. His reluctance to delegate would have crystallised into certain refusal if he perceived the people below him as inefficient, and this is exactly how he seemed to view the ICS at one point.

The main point to be examined, then, is not how he perceived the ICS, nor what course of action his perceptions led him to take, but what methods he used to combat 'inefficiency' when he found it. This was also the dominant theme in his early interactions with Madras and Bombay. As Viceroy the people from the ICS he came into extensive contact with were senior administrators, the heads of provinces and departments. The following section examines how Curzon functioned in the Viceregal office with respect to dealing with two of his Lieutenant Governors—a study in contrast between the Punjab and the United Provinces.

POWER UNSHEATHED: CURZON VS. MACKWORTH YOUNG

Since this book examines the extent to which Curzon was able to exercise unfettered power in his drive to streamline Indian administration, one aspect of this chapter examines what happened when he really did exercise roughshod power, when creating the North-West Frontier Province in 1901. While the creation of this province was not initiated by Curzon, in pushing it through, he alienated forever Sir William Mackworth Young, an ICS officer of almost forty years' standing, who was Lieutenant Governor of the Punjab, out of which the NWFP was lopped off. It is interesting to note that in the other province whose boundaries he redrew, i.e., Bengal, the incumbent governor was in full agreement with him, yet it was that which was reversed under popular pressure six years later.

Mackworth Young (1840–1924) had joined the Punjab cadre in 1864, and exemplified the stereotypical attitudes of that cadre.[11] Curzon thought that while he was conscientious, he could not divorce the personal from the political and took every act that went against the Punjab Government as a slur upon his abilities. He had opposed Curzon in 1900 over the Punjab Land Alienation Act (though this may have been inspired by professional jealousy of Charles Rivaz, who was the main proponent of the act, rather than defiance of Curzon, who played a comparatively minor role in the passing of this legislation), and this possibly worsened the slight he felt when he was not consulted over the creation of the NWFP. It would appear too that he was not backed by any of his own frontier specialists, purely because they all thought they would have the chance of a chief commissionership when the new province was created, and hence backed Curzon; a case of being disenfranchised by his superiors, and facing insubordination from administrators ranked below him—by this point he was, after all, the head of the Punjab province. The final blow came when Curzon decided to shift Punjab's summer capital from Simla to Ambala.[12]

In 1900, however, it was the Punjab Land Alienation Act which bitterly divided the Punjab Secretariat. The basic aim of this act was to remedy 'the gradual transfer of ownership of the soil from its natural lords,' the 'Musalman tribes,' to 'astute . . . Hindu traders and bankers,'[13] in short, to prevent land being alienated. While it had much impact upon future Indian political development in the region, and is still in force, it will here be analysed for the divergences and differences it threw up among the governing British. This is because, while Curzon was the force that pushed the Bill through to law, as demonstrated in Chapter Six, the Punjab Land Alienation Bill also demonstrates how Curzon's was not a Viceroyalty that relied on one-sided policy initiatives from the top down. It was the ICS that was primarily responsible for bruiting the idea of the Act and Curzon's senior ICS officials, principally in this case Charles Rivaz, exercised a palpable influence on him and they, and Curzon, were in turn affected by the political and economic climate of contemporary Britain and India.

The Punjab Land Alienation Bill was an idea that had been doing the rounds of the secretariat for a quarter of a century before Curzon came to India. It was one instance where the ICS could truly be said to be an originator of policy. The idea had first been officially propounded by S.S. Thorburn. By Curzon's time, the main players, all of them past or future governors of the Punjab, were Denzil Ibbetson; Home Member, Charles Rivaz; Dennis Fitzpatrick at the India Office; Mackworth Young, the incumbent Governor of the Punjab; and Curzon himself. For much legislation passed by him, Curzon was a link in a chain who 'stimulated certain general trends in opinion than repressing them.'[14] In this case, Curzon mostly took his cue from Sir Charles Rivaz, then Home Member, and worked closely with him to pass the Bill. It helped that Denzil Ibbetson, for whom Rivaz was filling in as Home Member on the Viceroy's Council, shared his views about the sort of legislation desirable to contain land alienations. Both had long experience of the conditions in the Punjab, and with inputs (albeit hostile ones) from Fitzpatrick in London, Curzon could well afford to sideline Mackworth Young, as he had access to some of the most prominent experts of the age.

It was in part due to this collaboration that Curzon offered the Lieutenant Governorship of the Punjab to Rivaz at the close of Mackworth Young's term, because, as he observed to Rivaz, he would 'have the congenial responsibility of carrying into effect legislative changes, in the evolution of which you have borne a conspicuous part.'[15] This was the same line of thought that would see the India Office pass over Ampthill as Curzon's successor because he did not care to mask his disapproval of Kitchener's military reforms. As demonstrated below, while the Punjab Land Alienation Act itself demonstrated a departure from traditional liberalism and *laissez-faire*,[16] the manner of its passing was marked by inter-departmental negotiations and recriminations that were reflective of the long standing divergences opinion over policy that characterised the Indian Empire. It also reflected the ICS' ultimate dependence upon the Viceroy; had Curzon chosen to be convinced by the opponents of the Bill, it might have languished within departmental files until the arrival of his successor. This also opens up the possibility of sections of the ICS, or indeed of any administrative department, advocating their viewpoint before a superior who might be inclined to regard it favourably to fast track their most cherished projects. The Punjab school of government, within itself, nursed deep divisions, a situation that presented as many obstacles as freeways to passing legislation to any incumbent Viceroy. But why did Curzon, so against special pleading when it came from the Indians, assent to the Punjab Land Alienation Bill? His stance cannot be solely attributed to the championing of the Bill in one form or the other by the (admittedly formidable) trio of Ibbetson, Rivaz, and Fitzpatrick—he is known to have snubbed Lawrence's observation that the Indians would welcome a hint that their future might be self-determined.

The Punjab Land Alienation Act of 1900 and the Co-operative Societies Act of 1904, it has been suggested, illustrate a novel attitude in the British Government of India.[17] D.A. Low suggests that in the late nineteenth century there was a marked reaction to the reforming tendencies which had been prevalent in its governing circles in the first half of the century. The shift was centred upon the proposition that society was more fragile than had earlier been allowed and that checks should therefore be imposed upon the workings of the social order so as to ensure that liberty should not become licence. The obvious fear was that the flower of the yeomanry might rise up in rebellion; a less immediate concern was that the yeomanry might totally cease to exist. These were concerns Curzon could sympathise with. The motives behind the Bill also dovetailed neatly with the aims of the reforms Curzon himself had initiated; the economic motive fit in with his efforts at improving the state of the agrarian population, and the political one appealed to his efforts to improve the security of India, internally and externally.

Thus duly convinced by the arguments put forth by the Punjab ICS arguing for the necessity of the measure, Curzon, as seen above, wrote to Hamilton urging support for the measure. Hamilton went to the extent of ensuring that Alfred Lyall was not present the day it was passed by the Council; Dennis Fitzpatrick did not oppose it, in this instance disproving the theory that the old India Hands on the Council were merely there to block legislation that ran contrary to the methods of governance *they* had preferred.

* * *

But, despite the Punjab Land Alienation Act being one of the few reforms of Curzon's Viceroyalty which were the result of collaboration with the ICS and almost universally approved, Mackworth Young, governor of Punjab, was against it. In this he was merely echoing the example of his predecessor Fitzpatrick, but whereas Fitzpatrick's rejection of the bill was based on that fact that he wanted to prohibit permanent alienations to non-agriculturalists alone, Young objected to the Bill in totality, as he favoured free-trade. As will be seen in Chapter Six, he attempted to introduce a protégé of his into the committee set up to investigate the Bill. Curzon successfully foiled this by introducing a handpicked Indian to neutralise this, but by then he had already come to distrust Mackworth Young, further evidence of his astute man-management skills.

It was probably this that made Curzon disinclined to consult Mackworth Young about the NWFP. Geographic determinism and historical geography were the major impetuses behind the creation of the NWFP. As far as the severance from the Punjab was concerned, the creation of NWFP would seem to have been a right move given the differences in geography and ethnicity between the inhabitants of Bannu, Kohat, Dera Ismail Khan and the Punjab. The well-farmed plains of the Punjab, though a famous recruitment ground for the Indian Army, were a sharp contrast to rugged mountain habitat of the 'magnificent Samsons' of the border. Lytton in 1877 had attempted to coalesce the entire region of what is now modern Pakistan into a single administrative block;[18] Curzon, recognising the differences between the Punjab and the other provinces, decided to modify Lytton's plan and create a province composed of just the frontier districts—which then came under the aegis of the Punjab Government—whose government would report directly to the Government of India. But he declined to consult the governor from whose province these territories were to be abstracted.

Curzon was not alone in wanting to exclude Mackworth Young from the deliberations; Secretary of State George Hamilton, who enthusiastically backed the frontier plan, also backed the plan to *not* involve the Punjab Government. Curzon asked Hamilton for his view about the 'necessity or desirability' of consulting them, as he thought Mackworth Young was 'naturally slow, very sensitive, very disputatious, rather long-winded,'[19] and his objections would slow down the process of reform. Hamilton thereupon wrote to Curzon that,

> any proposal that you make by which the Punjab Government will permanently be deprived of its present control over relations with frontier tribes, will be opposed in this Council. But the proposal is of such a character that it must be the Cabinet, and not the Council, who decide whether or not it shall be adopted. I think, therefore, it would be better not to consult Mackworth Young in the first instance. You would have to overrule him by putting on one side his objections. He, or the officials connected with the Punjab Government, are perfectly certain to write to certain Members of Council here. They will pick up their ears, and be on the *qui vive* as regards any despatch which comes home, and they will in anticipation have formed opinions hostile to your proposals. If under such conditions I refer your proposal to the Cabinet, it would look as if I did so because I wished, by this extraneous method, to override the opposition of my Council. On the other hand, if the proposal comes straight home, and I refer it at once to the Cabinet, the Council would by constitution acquiesce in the decision of the Cabinet without demur.[20]

The above not only illustrates how Hamilton felt about Mackworth Young—his opinion concurred with that of Curzon's—but also how Hamilton and Curzon colluded in matters of Indian polity, as discussed in Chapter Two.[21] In this instance they very successfully managed to outmanoeuvre both the Indian Civil Service and the Council of India. This is one instance where India would really seem to have been governed by confidential correspondence between the Secretary of State and the Viceroy. Because Curzon and Hamilton got on so well, they could decide which bit of political machinery to use and manipulate when it suited them, proof of the instrumentality of inter-personal relations in high politics. This was not repeated with Brodrick, costing Curzon, ultimately, the Viceroyalty. It also highlights exactly how rife political expediency was, because while Hamilton always insisted that due respect must be shown to the Council, he did not hesitate to cast aside his own principles when the exigencies so demanded it. This might also pinpoint to the fact that Curzon was in fact largely right about the 'crabbed' character of the Council, but, conterminously, the Council would also have been justified had they complained about being bypassed in a sneaky manner. Finally, this episode also highlights the fact that this was one instance where Curzon's expertise of Asian affairs (more precisely frontier affairs) helped him get his own way as it was what persuaded his fellow co-sharers of powers that he knew best when he proposed the creation of the NWFP. This was something the ICS was not heavily involved in; the legendary frontier administrators had mostly been soldiers. Curzon's knowledge gave him an edge over Mackworth Young.

Of course, this also shows one instance where Curzon was in collusion with Hamilton, and also that Hamilton fully realized that the India Council could be wilfully obstructive, especially when it came to protecting their 'fellow' Indian Civilian's interests. Hence this comment of Hamilton's is extremely telling, indicative as it is on the many implications that can be read from it in terms of Curzon's style of governance. But Hamilton's fears about backstairs political negotiations between the India Council and ICS were not unfounded; lobbying for posts and airing grievances against superiors through the Council was a practice of long-standing, as demonstrated above, and Curzon later illustrated how Mackworth Young planned to use it:

> It appears that when the first rumours [about the carving out of the NWFP] got about, Mackworth Young assured all his men that they need not be in the least alarmed; that his party at the India Office was quite sufficiently strong to defeat any such project. . . . When the acceptance of the scheme by His Majesty's Government was finally announced . . . they all turned round, said they had been deceived by their Lieutenant Governor, and that the least he could do would be to resign. When he showed no intention of doing this, their disgust was enhanced. . . .[22]

But on what grounds did Young oppose the creation of the NWFP? As discussed below, his objection as to the mode of creating it, without involving him, is certainly attributable to feeling disempowered, but what was his administrative justification for the stand he took? To what extent was this, in fact, bound up with his professional insecurities, if any?

He laid out his most weighty objections in a memo to Curzon, opining firstly that:

'The method of settling this long-debated frontier question by detaching from the Punjab administration and control the trans-frontier tracts politically connected with it . . . has been arrived at without any opinions from the Punjab Government having been asked.' This, as can be seen, was his main grievance. He continued that he had 'given my reasons for objecting to this procedure, and the Government of India have dealt with my objections. I have not thought it proper'—a conscious affirmation of his subordinate status and the constraints this imposed upon him 'or necessary to make any rejoinder . . . [but] I feel bound to indicate in some detail the dangers and drawbacks of the plan.'[23]

That Curzon had gone all the way back to Lytton, and as far as London, to seek opinions on the proposed province, undoubtedly alienated Mackworth Young more than anything else. When it became inevitable that the creation of the NWFP would, anyway, be seriously considered, he wrote to Curzon to ask Hamilton to suspend making a decision about it until he, Young, had had a chance of putting his views before the Secretary of State,[24] which he was not constitutionally privileged to do, but nonetheless tried to seek assurances from Walter Lawrence to the effect.[25] To this Curzon responded that there was no precedence of consulting local governors, that Lytton had never done so,[26] and that he was therefore not transgressing a constitutionalism by doing so:

If there had been good grounds for such a charge, I cannot but think that they would have been pointed out to me, possibly by the Secretary of State, who was aware of what I proposed to do, anyhow by those of my colleagues who have a much longer acquaintance with Indian constitutional procedure than I can claim.[27]

This is yet another instance where Curzon falls back upon the ICS and its deemed expertise in Indian administration to vindicate his stand regarding an administrative issue. This also throws up the sub-theme that the Punjab cadre were as sensitive to perceived slights to their authority within their boundaries, or with anything that concerned their administration, as the Bombay and Madras cadres; only this has not been highlighted by historians, or rather, has been passed off as bonding borne out of the experiences of the Mutiny. Re-tracing our steps to why Mackworth Young felt alienated, even insulted, however, it was, as Walter Lawrence reminiscenced, not just the wrenching away of a huge chunk of his province, nor the disregard for his authority, that engendered such feelings of disenfranchisement in Mackworth Young; it was the ruthlessness with which Curzon went about pointing out the necessity of the operation. As Lawrence noted,

> Curzon . . . never omitted a single detail in the elaboration of his plans . . . but as I had been in the Punjab I knew that the loss of this interesting charge would be bitterly resented by those who had so long watched and warded the passes into Afghanistan, and I was anxious that the wind should be tempered . . . I pointed out that he had proved his case and that some of the arguments were superfluous and might cause unnecessary pain to the Punjab Government. But he replied that a statesman should never omit an argument.[28]

From Curzon's point of view, of course, it was unfortunate that Mackworth Young should be in Punjab at that critical juncture; highlighting his 'incompetence' all the more starkly was the fact that his tenure was sandwiched between that of Sir Dennis Fitzpatrick and Sir Denzil Ibbetson, sterling administrators, both of whom went on to serve on the Viceroy's Council/India Council.

What added an extra dose of gall to Mackworth Young's post-NWFP campaign of subdued defiance was the participation of his wife; Curzon's views on women in public life were that they were best dissociated from it, and his Council appears to have thought along similar lines. Lady Young's intrusion upset ritualised protocol; when she offered to apologise for any offence her comments might have afforded the Viceroy, the law member of Curzon's Council, Thomas Raleigh, wrote to Lawrence that he did not know how exactly to proceed: 'My notion is, that when a married lady has to apologise, her husband ought to give the message. Sir M. has apologised on his own account . . .'[29]

From Curzon's point of view, thus, Mackworth Young was trying to hold on to a power he had (in Curzon's eyes) no claim to, because he was unfitted to handle it. This divorcing of power from *de jure* authority is one of the hallmarks of Curzon's Viceroyalty, but it is significant that when he spoke, he always justified his power on the grounds that he was an efficient Viceroy, and not just an efficient Asiatic affairs person who happened to be Viceroy.

In terms of administrative theory, Young's major objections were based on grounds of equitable governance and popular appeal:

> the severance of the five districts from the Province to which they have been attached since Sikh times will be unpopular with the chiefs and the people of the districts concerned . . . when these people come to realise that they have no right of appeal to Lahore, they will feel that their privileges under the British Government have been seriously curtailed.[30]

Young even cited a similar reasoning made by Sir Henry Davies, Lieutenant Governor in 1876, even as Curzon drew upon Lytton to provide backing for his plan. As to the 'people', Captain Roos-Keppel had already stated in May that year that,

> the only Hakim the Afridi knows is his Political Officer . . . of the higher authorities from whom that officer receives his orders he has little or no knowledge. Unless some radical change of policy be inaugurated with the formation of the new Province, it will probably be some years before the Afridi realises that there has been a change of system.[31]

That may well have been the case then, though Young was probably right about the long-term deleterious effects on the people. The new province was a 'non-regulation' province, with all power concentrated in the person of the single representative of the Government of India, making the administration necessarily paternalistic and authoritarian, even while being effective.[32] It adversely affected the political consciousness of the province, and its transition to modern democracy; though this, from Curzon's point of view, was probably an ideal outcome.

As noted above, the NWFP ran the gauntlet of public opinion and survives today; it was Bengal where 'the people' or at any rate a section of them, made their anti-redistribution feelings clearly known.

Young's other objection was that 'the miniature administration . . . will be much less efficient than that which now exists as part of a large Provincial organisation.' He also seemed to feel that, 'there will be a constant tendency in the new administration to play to the political gallery . . . the chief commissioner will be selected for his political, and not for his administrative, attainments.'[33] This, to an extent, was true. But like the Princely States, the frontier was an area where personal contact and the personal characteristics of the chief officer were instrumental in defining the character of the administration. All the warrant of precedence and the stress on hierarchy was nullified—that Curzon grasped this is testament to his skills of political perception, because it essentially went against the grain of his philosophy that it was the work that mattered, not who or how it was carried out. In fact, it was precisely to obviate administrative bureaucracy that the whole scheme had been instituted, a point which Young missed even as he refuted it.

Of course, while the chain of command was clearly one that caused Curzon great concern, it was because he felt it did not lead up to the proper apex. He said that 'the conduct of foreign affairs in India is vested in the Viceroy . . . Now in India foreign affairs . . . are [mostly] connected with the frontier tribes and problems.'[34] By this tendentious logic, the Viceroy as head of the central government, should have control of the frontier. By extension, according to Curzon, 'it is from the nature of things impossible for a Local Government to carry out a foreign policy which it neither originates in the first place nor is responsible for in the last, with the same influence, zeal or despatch as would the authors of the policy itself.'[35] As to distance from the frontier, he pointed out that for nearly half the year, both the central government and the Punjab Government were based at Simla. Young retaliated by pointing out that if the Viceroy were to be so closely connected with the day-to-day administration of the new province, whoever was appointed the Chief Commissioner of the new province would,

> feel so strongly the obligation of satisfying the Government of India in the Foreign Department in respect of his political duties, that with every desire to discharge his administrative duties efficiently, he will be unable to do so and will have to put them into commission by delegating them to his Lieutenants. An administration so carried on can never be a success.[36]

This sentiment, possibly calculated to arouse Curzon's detestation of delegating work, failed to change the Viceroy's views, and the NWFP was born.

A further blow came when Curzon, as a direct corollary of the creation of the NWFP, shifted the Punjab's summer capital out of Simla. Historically, the summer capital of the Punjab had been Murree, and it was only since the time of Lord Lytton that the Punjab Lieutenant Governor had begun to base himself at Simla due to the necessity of discussing frontier affairs with the Viceroy. In Curzon's opinion, now that the NWFP had been removed from the Punjab command, there remained no reason

> for the close propinquity, and indeed every reason against it. The Lieutenant Governor ought to be supreme in his own territories throughout the year. At Simla he is absolutely overshadowed by the Viceroy, and is almost a nonentity. The existence of two Secretariats side by side, at the opposite ends

of the same station, so far from producing harmony and rapidity of work, has precisely the opposite result. There is a good deal of stand aloofness, and sometimes positive friction, between the officers of the two Governments. If any dispute is proceeding between them, it is not always agreeable to their respective heads to be thrown into constant social contact.[37]

Young was to later bitterly subscribe to this view; but he did not initially view it that way. Propinquity to power held a powerful lure for the Punjab Government. They resented the fact that the Viceroy exercised maximum power in India only insofar as they were adversely affected by such exercise. But, in fact, members of the ICS had their methods and networks for bringing their colleagues to the notice of the Viceroy. For instance, Denzil Ibbetson and J.P. Hewett, in 1900, recommended Robert Nathan to Curzon for a CIE, because he had worked very hard during the plague. Nathan later became Curzon's private secretary.

In fact, the only thing Curzon consulted Mackworth Young about was the question of his successor. Curzon suggested Charles Rivaz, to which Young, possibly realising that the appointment was a foregone conclusion, gave his approval.[38] Mackworth Young came to epitomise all that Curzon found obnoxious about the ICS and that they felt the same about him. The next section examines the reverse: how a governor viewed with circumspection by his own cadre commanded an envied confidential relationship with the Viceroy.

CURZON AND SIR A.P. MACDONNELL

But Curzon's condemnation of the ICS could not have been wholly equivocal; after all, as we have seen, his private secretary was an ex-ICS man, he advocated the appointment of the Governors of Bombay and Madras from the ranks of the ICS, and he saw himself as a sort of 'head of the ICS'. Nowhere was this more strongly evident than in his dealings with A.P. MacDonnell, the Lieutenant Governor of the NWP and Oudh.

A.P. MacDonnell,[39] an Irishman who was a passionate supporter of Irish Home Rule, was the one Lieutenant Governor that Curzon wholly admired. An Irish Catholic from rural Connacht, it has been suggested that MacDonnell's boundless energy stemmed in part from a desire to obviate any expression of the ambiguity towards Irish appropriation of Imperial postings that might have hindered his career.[40] In fact a great proportion of senior administrators during Curzon's time were Irish.

The Curzon–MacDonnell relationship was uncomplicated and wholly revolved around matters of administration discussed in India itself and not constitutionalisms. Perhaps this was because of MacDonnell's own outsider status in the circles of British power, and also because he was a capable administrator. Curzon does not seem to have had a negative word for the Governor of the NWP and Oudh throughout. The secret of MacDonnell's success, he stated, was 'that he invariably sends for the local leaders, gets them on his side, makes them put their names to a document embodying his policy, and thus at the same time carries through what he wants, and remains free from attack.'[41] He backed MacDonnell's request for an extension in UP, which it seems was because he wanted to push through the Nagari resolution, telling Hamilton that, 'as a matter of fact, a movement is being widely organized in the Province—I admit by Natives—praying for a prolongation of his term: and I would rather comply before receiving the request than appear to yield to it at a later date.'[42] This is indicative of just how much Curzon wished to be seen as an administrator who would care nothing for Indian public opinion; the remark is also curious because it hints at a popularity enjoyed by the Governor; when in fact Curzon himself agreed that he would have to be passed over for the Governorship of Bombay because of his knack of alienating all those around him. It was chiefly for this reason, along with the Bombay cadre's hostility to outsiders, that he was passed over.[43] As Curzon noted, 'MacDonnell runs his own show with great ability (and great unpopularity).[44] The Nagari resolution, for example, was his own initiative, enabling the use of Hindi in government notifications because 'it has often occurred that an order in Urdu has been posted up in a village not a single soul in which could read it . . . [it was not made] because of any political considerations, but because of the over-whelming administrative necessity . . .'[45] Curzon merely gave it his unqualified approval, stating that he had 'not a doubt that . . . the declaration is one of equal liberality and justice.'[46]

In fact the Viceroy thought so highly of MacDonnell that he used his relationship with him to illustrate to the Secretary of State how he was being unfairly maligned for being allegedly harsh with his subordinate governors and other colleagues; 'that my standards are not impossible may, I think, be judged from the fact that, during the 1 ¾ years that I have been in India, I have not had one word of private or public disagreement with the strongest Governor [sic] now in the country, Sir A. MacDonnell.'[47] As Curzon was for once perceptive enough to realize, having the backing of this idiosyncratic administrator of long standing did much to dispel the myth of his inability to forge relationships with those in power with well-formed opinions not necessarily congruent to his own.

He warmly recommended MacDonnell for a seat in the India Council, perhaps as much with his own interests in view, as an affiliate there would reduce his frequent clashes with that antediluvian body:

> He would prove an invaluable recruit. His knowledge and ability are great: his subtlety is not inferior to his courage; and barring certain pronounced political inclinations [MacDonnell was a committed Home Ruler] which have a home [sic] rather than an Indian application, he is sufficiently Conservative for a Member of the Council of the Secretary of State.[48]

Of course, the fundamental reason that Curzon got on with MacDonnell was that he found him to be an efficient governor; their views on administrative affairs tended to tally. The strongest instance of this was the method of famine relief. Over the years, through independent studies of the Western Indian famine, their views on relief tended to converge, resulting finally in the report of the famine commission. The recommendations, which very emphatically de-emphasized the free distribution of largesse that had hitherto been the norm, bear the stamp of being formed by people who believed in controlled, tight administrative systems.[49] MacDonnell shared Curzon's views about making the peasant self-supporting. In consequence one of the chief concerns investigated by the Famine Commission was whether people on relief showed an inclination to be satisfied upon completion of enough work to garner them the minimum wage. To this the collector of Nasik answered in the affirmative; 'Yes, they loafed . . . we introduced a penal wage afterwards.'[50] The minimum wage was subsequently reduced by 25 per cent. But MacDonnell also shared Curzon's belief that the welfare of the lay peasantry was the British justification for being in India, and in consequence, the pair lobbied hard to ensure the passage of the Report in a form that would ensure security for the peasant. In August 1901 MacDonnell wrote to Curzon about a letter Sir Charles Crosthwaite on the India Council had written *him*; they differed over the method of land tenure. Crosthwaite was for 'abolishing the power of acquiring the tenant right, and for reducing all tenants to the level of holders for a term,' which MacDonnell feared would leave them exposed to arbitrary ejection. He threatened to resign, fulminating that,

> If the Secretary of State does not now accept the Bill, as approved by the Government of India, the conclusion is that he prefers to be guided by Crosthwaite's anti-tenant views, rather than by the views of the *men on the spot,* a turn of phrase sure to strike a sympathetic chord with the Viceroy; [emphasis added] which reconcile the interests of both parties. . . . If Crosthwaite's views prevail, I must leave to other hands the work of altering the Bill . . . Perhaps, to facilitate a decision, Your Excellency may think it worthwhile to inform Lord George Hamilton that Sir C. Crosthwaite's new idea in regard to ejectment [*sic*] has been fully considered here and rejected.[51]

Curzon promptly intimated this to Hamilton,[52] and was able to reassure MacDonnell that Hamilton had accepted the Bill as it stood.[53] As a matter of fact Hamilton had never pushed for alterations, telling Curzon that MacDonnell was 'unduly alarmed' about the fate of the Bill, even as he expressed the private view that legislation in the Empire was heavily skewed in favour of the tenant.[54] This demonstrates that not only was Curzon willing to back up his subordinates, but that he was also willing to indulge their protestations and gratify their personal wishes— MacDonnell was anxious that there should be no delay in passing the Bill as he was due to leave India shortly. As Viceroy he utilised the power of his office to function as an intermediary between the ICS and the Government in London, *viz.*, between the bureaucracy and the policy-makers, though these distinctions were fungible between the ICS and the India Office.

In the above instance one can discern parallels with Hamilton's backing, discussed above, of Curzon over the creation of the NWFP. Apart from the obvious patronage extended by the constitutional superiors in either case, what is noticeable is the transparency of the exchange between the parties concerned. That MacDonnell used Curzon as an intermediary to transmit his messages to London was exactly what Curzon wanted—and did not always get—in the case of Havelock, Ampthill, and Sandhurst.

But to say that Curzon and MacDonnell developed a healthy rapport because MacDonnell was intrinsically a governor whose style of functioning matched Curzon's expectations of how a model governor should function, and also happened to mirror Curzon's own style of communication, is being rather too harsh on the Presidency Governors. There were factors other than the inter-personal that were responsible for their efficient working relationship, the chief being the nature of the provincial administration. The United Provinces administrative cadre did not possess that healthy spirit of autonomy from Simla that the Bombay and—to a lesser degree—Madras governments did, owing to its historical circumstances. Had MacDonnell been governor at either of these places, it is probable that his Curzon-like drive for efficiency would have rubbed up the local secretariats the wrong way; certainly he was passed over as Governor of Bombay for this precise reason.[55] Curzon may have viewed Ampthill's pedantry as an annoying trait, but his stolid, yet steady approach ultimately worked wonders for the Madras administration, because he did not antagonise the Madras cadre by always pushing them on, something an enthusiastic, eager-beaver Governor would almost certainly have done. And neither the Madras nor the Bombay cadres *liked* being pushed about. It is true that MacDonnell was a valuable asset in that he managed to reassure Indian opinions, but local opinion in Bombay and Madras, was, again, of a very different character than in the United Provinces. Curzon's wishing for a dozen MacDonnells was one instance where his vision may have been flawed because he did not make it context-specific.

But by 1901 Curzon had fallen out with MacDonnell, complaining to Hamilton about the manner in which MacDonnell had prohibited the Talukdars of Oudh from contributing to the Viceroy's Victoria Memorial Scheme, and had instructed them instead to subscribe towards the North-Western Provinces' Local Fund.[56] To this Hamilton replied that Curzon might hint to MacDonnell that, 'running counter to the Viceroy in an unreasonable spirit is not likely to increase his chances of getting an appointment to the Secretary of State's Council, as the latter official is naturally influenced in his selections by the opinions of the Viceroy as to the capacity for work and cooperation of the retired officials who come home.'[57] But Curzon was not the person to entertain a grudge and told Hamilton he should certainly place MacDonnell on the India Council, as befitted a man of 'such great ability'.[58] This was obviously a blatant attempt on the part of the home establishment to keep out someone with undesirable political views, using his former patron as a cat's paw; a hint of how scruples would be cast aside in the Kitchener affair. MacDonnell, in any event, left India in 1903. And Sandhurst's successor in Bombay was Lord Northcote, and not Alfred Lyall, who had also been mooted. This was an instance where Curzon's consideration of people's opinions before taking an action erred on the wrong side of caution. The people, if not the government, of the Bombay Presidency would have welcomed MacDonnell. In 1903 the Bombay press even suggested he might be a good successor to Curzon:

Sir Anthony [*sic*] MacDonnell is well known in India for his sympathy towards the people, as well as his sound common sense and administrative capacity; and if he returns to India as Viceroy he will have a hearty welcome from the Indian people and it will also be an honour to the ICS.[59]

Of course, no ICS man after John Lawrence ever became Viceroy. However, the study of the Curzon–MacDonnell relationship is crucial to dispelling some of the myths surrounding Curzon's ability to forge mutually constructive working relationships. His biographer Dilks attributes his ultimately warm relationship with Ampthill and Lamington to the fact that both were junior to him in age and experience— presumably, any dialogue over matters of administration with these two was wholly dominated by Curzon.[60] While Chapter Three has demonstrated how Ampthill was certainly not intimidated by Curzon, the fact that Curzon was able to establish an equable relationship with MacDonnell demonstrates that Curzon *was* able to convince the senior ICS of his bona fides.

A comparative study of MacDonnell, Mackworth Young and their very different rapports with Curzon throws up many interesting reflections. These respective personalities had come up through the same system within a few years of each other, albeit in different provinces. Yet they aroused very different reactions from Curzon. The very qualities Curzon might respect enterprising spirit, a certain lack of disregard for bureaucratic rules, could be taken too far, in his estimation, especially if they were used to shoehorn what he perceived as unjustified advantages for one province over another. Curzon's dislike of governors standing up too enthusiastically for their provinces is not understandable in the light of his failure to see why the India Office might have sought to curb what they saw as his reckless championing of Indian interests over Imperial ones.

A.P. MacDonnell was at the fag-end of his career in the ICS when Curzon arrived in India; the rising star then was Harcourt Butler, who had joined the ICS in 1890.[61] Butler, who wrote extensively to Richmond Ritchie, forms an interesting counterpoint to MacDonnell's analysis; he also appears to have subscribed to all the stereotypical ideologies attributed to the British in India; as a representative official, his views are important. Butler thought Curzon was insufficiently accommodating towards the Indians, and shared the view that by denouncing the Congress Curzon was giving it a fillip.

Maconochie gives an insight into how Curzon actually worked, as opposed to merely stating how he single-handedly attempted to get work done. Here he is, talking about how R.C. Dutt's charge that famines were caused by excessive taxation was rebutted:

> The first step taken was an examination by the department concerned . . . Mr Holderness took up the Zamindari Provinces and handed the Raiyatwari over to me . . . whatever the use to Government of my investigations, their pursuit was an education to me, and when I left Simla I knew more than most . . . Mr Dutt's criticisms were forwarded to the Local Governments and their replies invited. The final result was the resolution of the Governor General in Council, No. 1, dated January 16, 1902, which, with its appendices, contains a complete exposition of the policy of Government.[62]

The provincial governorships were only one means by which the ICS and Curzon actively collaborated in the formation of polity. The other was the Viceroy's Council. In Curzon's time, a third avenue was instituted by which the ICS could have a say in influencing the Viceroy; the office of Private Secretary to the Viceroy. When Curzon appointed Walter Lawrence as his Private Secretary, the job consisting of being essentially a buffer between the Viceroy and the masses, including 'filtering, screening and mediating',[63] it was a departure from precedent. Lawrence himself, for reasons above personal modesty, demurred. As he noted, 'up to this time, the private secretaries had been selected from England.' Lawrence himself was an ex-ICS man who gave up a pension with the Duke of Bedford to return to India, because 'it seemed to me that it would help a Viceroy to have with him someone who knew at any rate the puzzling terms and technicalities with which the Indian administration bristles.'[64] And of these, as Gilmour has noted, there were very many.

Lawrence might have been right, but not everyone thought along these lines of logic. Lansdowne's ex-Private Secretary wrote to Curzon expressing a totally contrarian view to the one held by Lawrence: 'Don't take an Indian Civilian. They are all too closely bound up in the country. An outsider will be far more useful, particularly one who knows English official and parliamentary routine, and the exigencies of party government.'[65] This might have been true, especially in the light of Curzon's contretemps with the Home Government, but since Lawrence left in 1903, and Curzon's next secretary too was an 'Indian Civilian', the theory remained untested throughout the Kitchener Affair. But the Private Secretary did increasingly become a focal point of reference for those civilians wanting to get a message or a plea across to the Viceroy, all the more so because Lawrence was seen as being rather more approachable than Curzon. It set a precedent; after Lawrence went back to England, the other two Private Secretaries, Robert Nathan, and John Ontario Miller, were both drawn from the ICS.

* * *

Interestingly, while the ICS, or its ex-members, should have stuck up for Curzon's suggestion that recruiting the Governors of Bombay and Madras from their ranks might be a good thing, it was an ex-ICS member who proposed extending the system of bringing in external persona to other provinces. In 1901, Alfred Lyall, otherwise so conservative when it came to sanctioning new plans, suggested that it might be worthwhile to make someone Lieutenant Governor of the Punjab who had not spent his career in that province, given that, 'the true-bred Punjabee . . . is strongly prepossessed in favour of certain views and a certain system.'[66] Of course, breadth of vision was also a reason why no Viceroy or Governor of Bombay and Madras was ever chosen from the ICS if other options were available. And it is possible that inter-provincial rivalry was confined to Bombay and Madras, or even largely existed only among the Bombay cadre. But, as seen in Chapter Three, Curzon himself had reservations about the extreme overhauling the administrative system in the presidencies would require were the post of Governor to be made over to an ICS man. From this one may conclude that Curzon's views about the ICS, and therefore his relationship with them were influenced, in short, by a mixture of social class, official equations forged in the traditions of British India, and also regional attitudes within India. What is surprising, in light of the fact that many biographers have pointed to his extraordinary administrative skills, why he did not himself join the ICS. The explanation that springs most readily to mind is that of social class; people of Curzon's relatively aristocratic and titled background would not enrol themselves among the ranks of the bureaucracy. His love of ordering polity is another reason; the ICS was not an originator of polity. A final factor is his romanticization of the office of Viceroy, which fused as it did the concepts of stewardship of India, links with the Crown, and an acknowledged place in the line-up of British ministerial designations.

CURZON AND THE VICEROY'S COUNCIL[67]

Because Walter Lawrence was an ex-ICS man, he was also involved in the deliberations of the Viceroy's Council. This body, a handpicked team that functioned somewhat like a modern Cabinet, was the other major way in which Curzon interacted with the ICS, and this was, in a way, more fraught than his relationships with either Mackworth Young or MacDonnell, because the Viceroy's Council's every move was watched by observers at the India Office for signs of excessive subordination or otherwise to the Viceroy.

A great part of the authority of the Viceroy stemmed from the fact that he was, *ex-officio*, the head of the governing Council of India. As an old India hand noted at the height of the Kitchener dispute,

> The statute is perfectly clear that . . . the superintendence, direction and control of the whole civil and military government shall be vested in a Governor General and Counsellors [sic] . . . no one of these counsellors has the right to separately administer any department. If the order which he alone proposes is issued by the Secretary to Government, it issues as an order

of the Governor General in Council, and derives its authority from their corporate acceptance of it. At the same time . . . a process of centralization has been going on in the last few years [and] the personal term 'Viceroy' has figured in despatches as it has never done before . . . [but] it ought to be understood that the law provides for one control only, that of the Governor General in Council; and less friction would be caused if those words were more frequently used in official literature. . . . The Governor General in Council alone directs and controls.[68]

And Lee-Warner was not even pro-Curzon, quite the opposite!

For members of the ICS, of course, being on the Council was one way by which they could express direct power. Hence this section also seeks to explore the relationship between the Viceroy's Council and the ICS. How did the ICS see the Council; did they view them as a link to the Viceroy or as former comrades-in-arms who had gone over to the other side? Evan Maconochie's father-in-law, Denzil Ibbetson, was on the Council, and Maconochie notes how he knew a lot of people around. How did the Council see its role? The interaction between the India Council and the ICS (their possible feeding off each other) has been documented, but the Viceroy's Council has been largely overlooked. Obviously a place on the Council could be given to someone who had risen through the ranks of the covenanted civil service, and this was always the case, except in the case of the Law Members. Yet, while competition for Governorships was rife, the ICS does not seem to have attached the same importance to a seat on the Viceroy's Council, and this section examines the reasons for it. The Council itself was not necessarily composed of people from the ICS; in fact, there was a tendency to strike a balance between Civilians and men brought out from Home.

During Curzon's term in office, the members of his Council (and the army Commanders-in-Chief, who *did not* have a seat on the Council) were as follows:[69]

Table 1

Members of Curzon's Council

Name	Portfolio	Term of Office
Clinton Dawkins	Finance	1899
Sir Edward Law	Finance	1900–1905
Sir E.H.H. Collen	Military	1898–1901
Sir Edmond Elles	Military	1902–1905
Sir Thomas Raleigh	Law	1899–April 1904
Sir H. Erle Richards	Law	April 1904–1905
Sir A.T. Arundel	Public Works	1898–1905
Sir Charles Rivaz	Home	1899–1902
Sir Denzil Ibbetson	Home	1902–1905
Sir William Lockhart	Commander-in-Chief	1898–1900
Sir Power Palmer	Commander-in-Chief	1900–1903
Earl Kitchener	Commander-in-Chief	1903–1905

Of these, only Richards, Rivaz, and Ibbetson were ICS men. For the most part, Curzon appears to have regarded his council as a collection of curiosities. Denzil Ibbetson was one of the few officers he admired, and this admiration was reciprocated; Ibbetson (and J.P. Hewett) offered to resign along with Curzon and renounce their pensions in 1905. Ibbetson was sensitive to the changes of mood among his colleagues and the Council, and Curzon once wrote to him that he had 'such confidence in your advice (though this sounds rather a paradox) that I prefer your first thoughts to your second.'[70] But even Ibbetson (like A.P. MacDonnell, the other Governor whom Curzon expressed approval of) did not escape a few reproaches; in March 1904 we find him writing to Curzon asking to be excused for not having gotten through two outstanding cases due to ill-health and his wife's absence—perhaps the wrong excuses to plead before Curzon.[71] As to the rest, he noted in 1901: '[Charles] Rivaz does his work . . . with sobriety, but without a spark either of enthusiasm or initiative. Collen and I now languish in each other's arms. Trevor is marking time till the day of release dawns . . .'[72]

However, the Council had several diligent members upon it, even if they never quite matched Curzon's mental agility. One of these was the first Law Member, Sir Thomas Raleigh, a man of 'cloistered appearance and sequestered habits,'[73] who went on to produce a compendium of Curzon's Viceregal speeches. Despite this, Curzon described him as,

> although a man of fine intellect and much ability, [he] is essentially an Oxford Don, and in no sense a leader of men . . . he cannot . . . drive anything along . . . What we want in our Legal Member is a lawyer of good abilities and experience, who can speak and debate well, who can conduct difficult Bills through Committee, and who knows sufficient jurisprudence to save us in our ordinary business from legal mistakes . . . in consequence of the great names that have been connected with it in the past, it is both desirable and necessary to select someone of standing and reputation . . .[74]

Though Curzon did concede that he was useful to have around, and very handy for odd jobs,[75] Raleigh was eventually succeeded by Sir H. Erle Richards, who, like everyone else in the later stages of the Curzon Viceroyalty, devoted much of his time to cogitating over the constitutionalisms or otherwise of Kitchener's various demands for reform.

The other outstanding Councillor was Clinton Dawkins, the Finance Member for a year in 1899. During his term he did much to make the path of free enterprise easier in India; until Curzon and Dawkins,

> the attitude of the Government of India towards men anxious to invest their brains and their capital in India was that of the bulldog towards the burglar . . . Mr Dawkins, who possessed a wide knowledge not only of Government finance, but also of the great business world, pleaded strongly for a more liberal policy, and this attitude was warmly welcomed by the Viceroy . . .[76]

He then went back to become a merchant banker in the City, but continued to write politically insightful letters to the Viceroy throughout his tenure. By contrast, his successor, Edward Law, was not a man whom

Curzon warmed to; partly because he had no Indian experience and no knowledge of unique Indian situations.

The Home Member was perhaps the most important person on the Council, and it is notable that both the incumbents during Curzon's time were from the Punjab—revealing of the preponderance of the North in the mental landscape of the Raj. In the context of this thesis, it is worthwhile considering how having two influential Punjab civilians on his Council helped Curzon gain the support he needed from that body to counter the incumbent Punjab governor's protests over the Land Alienation Act, and how being on the Council helped these two— Ibbetson and Rivaz—gain the Viceroy's ear.

Curzon was acutely sensitive to the fact that the people on his Council were, essentially, from the ICS and not the governing elite. He shot down Brodrick's speculations as to whether their annual pay of £5300 could be improved upon, saying that it was 'ample for a promoted Civilian and quite sufficient for the class of man whom we get from home.'[77]

The Commander-in-Chief was not, of course, a member of the Council, in fact, it was the fact that the Military Member acted there in his stead that was the trigger that ended Curzon's time in office. This illustrates the importance attached to a seat on the Council, which was a sure shot way of guaranteeing the attention of the Viceroy. It would be all too easy for a Councillor to acquiesce in a Viceroy's proposal with the hope of gaining either a Governorship or a seat on the India Council after completion of his term. This was why the Viceroy's Council, while not figuring prominently in Indian public life, attracted a great deal of attention from the India Office during the politically turbulent years of the Curzon Viceroyalty. This was probably why St. John Brodrick as Secretary of State protested violently when Denzil Ibbetson resigned from the Council in 1904 to become temporary governor of the Punjab—he could not hold both posts simultaneously. Brodrick wrote of the disapproval of the India Council at this: 'here on the [India]

Council they attach the greatest possible importance to any change in *personnel,* though I am afraid you would not consider that this would make much difference to the course of business. . . .'[78] Ibbetson was one of the most prominent ICS men of his time, and Brodrick evidently thought Curzon was trying to remove what might have been a dissident voice on his Council. He would not, of course, have known of the warm working relationship shared by Curzon and Ibbetson. It is possible that Brodrick was trying to express his own views through the media of the India Council. He had touched upon the matter the month before, when it becomes clear that he actually professed to be concerned about the perception of a weakened Council in the eyes of the world:

> the present composition of the Council, with 4 men all brought in during the past year, is one that gives no authority outside to their decisions other than that which attaches to the prestige of the Viceroy, and to yourself in particular. . . . The unanimity of your Council is represented to be that of a body of men, so many of whom are personally dependent . . . on the Viceroy. It would have helped me very much in fighting for the decisions of your Council if there had been more outside influence.[79]

Curzon refuted this. 'I do not myself think that Members of Council are any more dependent upon the Viceroy than Cabinet ministers at Home are upon the Prime Minister, or the Members of your Council upon you.' He further sought to remind Brodrick of the slights he felt the Government of India had anyway been dealt: 'I do not remember that while [Ibbetson] has been with us, any greater weight has been attached to our advice than will probably be the case in the future. He also strove to dismiss claims that by putting his 'own men' in he was benefiting them in any undue ways:

> 'the utmost that the Viceroy can ever do is make a member of his Council a Lieutenant Governor . . . in 9 cases out of 10 . . . a man is marked out for succession to the chief post of a province in a manner so conspicuous that the Viceroy has not much influence upon the course of events . . .' and finally he rebutted the claim that his Council was dependent on him;

'Councillors here seem to me to be quite as independent as any similar
Committee I have seen elsewhere . . .'[80]

But it soon became clear that it was not the turnover, or the relative
inexperience at that level of the then new members of Council, that
Brodrick was concerned about. Basically, he did not want the Viceroy's
Council to be composed of Indian Civilians: 'I have been most reluctant
to complete your Council from officials serving in India, however
distinguished. Honestly I think you want new blood, and an
independence which no man who has been brought up under the Indian
system can altogether feel.'[81] What Curzon cared about, however, was
competence, not where the person came from. It is probable that
Brodrick thought planting the Council with people fresh from England
would give him direct access to the Viceroy's methods of administration,
but too many such incidences might have provoked an outcry from the
ICS at what they would have rightly seen as another denial of their rights
to partake in decision making for India. It is also not clear why Brodrick
should have felt that Indian civilians would be complaisant with
Curzon's ideas, because Curzon never ceased complaining about their
intransigence. Nor did the ICS go overboard in proclaiming their
enthusiasm for him, even if they did acknowledge his organisational
efficiency. As a matter of fact, if Curzon was right, they used the
influence of their ex-colleagues, now on the India Council, to attempt
a negation of the Viceroy's reforms.

Thus, trying to bring in more men from England to serve upon the
Council would definitely have caused mutterings from the ICS-for them,
it would have meant the removal of access to high government. Within
the Indian Empire, proximity to the Viceregal machine was considered
a sure-fire method of being noticed, promotions, and a permanent post
in Simla. This was one of the reasons the Punjab provincial government
did not want to give up sharing its seat with the Central government
at Simla and move to Ambala. As Curzon wrote to Brodrick about
it, 'Rivaz (ex-Punjab civilian and member of the Viceroy's Council
before he went back to the Punjab as Lieutenant Governor) is . . .

influenced . . . by his civilians, who think they will not get so many chances of promotions, when they are not in immediate contact with the Government of India.' But this argument only served to strengthen Curzon's justification for the removal of the Punjab Government: 'if there is anything in the belief, [it] is of course a strong reason for the change, since the Punjab enjoys an advantage denied to other Local Governments.'[82] It is apparent from this that members of the Council were certainly not disinterested yes men looking to further their chances of Lieutenant Governorships by being the Viceroy's sycophants; indeed, quite the reverse.

Nor did they hesitate in taking an independent line when they thought fit to do so; most notably when Ampthill was presiding as Viceroy and they did not agree with him (or Curzon) about the necessity for opposing Kitchener's proposal for army reforms. But other than that, it was really not possible for the Council to diverge sharply from the Viceroy because Indian polity was generally consensually formulated after feedback from the provincial administrators concerned; and major legislative changes were often in the pipeline for years before a decision was reached, which would have given everyone a chance to air their views and perceive the direction the debate was taking. The Viceroy was not a top-down formulator of policy, though he may have been a strong initiator; as seen in the matter of the governorships, the machine had a way of functioning upon its own momentum, even if Lawrence and Curzon thought that momentum was one of half-speed.

But it is clear that Curzon attached a lot of importance to having a qualitatively sound Viceroy's Council, much more certainly than he did to that other advisory body, the India Council. But this made sense; the Viceroy's Council had its specialisms very clearly defined and as such had the potential to back up a Viceroy magnificently. Further, the people on the Council were currently serving officers in various capacities and hence could be relied on to be in touch with the contemporary scenario. Finally, as observed above, a Council that could be proven to be independent would help his cause in London.

While the Viceroy's Council is often seen as being complaisant with Curzon's wishes and uniform in its action, the lack of dissension being held up as the result of a disallowance of free expression, it may have been because they were all of the same mind, broadly speaking.

In conclusion, while there was no deliberate nexus between the ICS and the Viceroy's Council, or even the Council of India in London, it is entirely understandable that once civil servants secured a place on any of these, they might be expected to utilise it to promote their long held administrative schemes to the incumbent Viceroy. As observed, these councils offered a means of access to the highest echelons of power, which were otherwise not open to an individual not from an appropriate socio-political background. Curzon needed the ICS to implement his plans, and they needed him to voice their plans to the governmental structure.

Thus far, the thesis has explored Curzon's relations with the civil administration of India. The next chapter takes on the Indian Army.

Notes

1. Penderel Moon, *The British Conquest and Dominion of India*, (London: Duckworth, 1989).
2. Edwardes, *High Noon of the Raj*, p. 257.
3. Philip Mason, *The Men Who Ruled India*, (London: Jonathan Cape, 1985), pp. 265, 268.
4. Khalid bin Sayeed, *Pakistan: The Formative Phase*, (Karachi: OUP, 1968).
5. George Curzon, *Speech at the Indian Civil Service Dinner Club*, 08 July 1910, Curzon Papers, Mss Eur F112/592, pp. 56–7.
6. For a full database, see Shigematsu Shinji (ed.), *ICS: Database of ICS Members, 1790–1905* (Nagoya: University of Nagoya, 1984).
7. Judith Brown, 'Imperial Façade: Some Constraints upon and Contradictions in the British Position in India, 1919–1935'. *Transactions of the Royal Historical Society*, 5:26 (1976): p. 38.
8. Lawrence, *The India We Served*, pp. 223–44.
9. Evan Maconochie, *Life in the Indian Civil Service*, (London: Chapam and North, 1926), p. 110.
10. Curzon to Hamilton, 21 May 1902, Curzon Papers, Mss Eur F111/161.

11. *Oxford Dictionary of National Biography*, available from www.oxforddnb.com, accessed 14 January 2008.

12. There is no biography of Mackworth Young, but this section draws heavily upon the entry in the *Oxford Dictionary of National Biography*, (Katherine Prior), available at http://www.oxforddnb.com/veiw/printable/37081, accessed 18 January 2008.

13. S.S. Thorburn, *Musalmans & Moneylenders in the Punjab*, (New Delhi: Mittal Publications, 1984 [1886]), p. 1.

14. P.H.M. van den Dungen, *The Punjab Tradition: Influence and Authority in Nineteenth Century India*, (London: George Allen & Unwin, 1972), p. 280.

15. Curzon to Rivaz, 23 August 1901, Curzon Papers, Mss Eur F111/204.

16. Van den Dungen, *The Punjab Tradition*, p. 279.

17. D.A. Low, 'Laissez-Faire and Traditional Rulership in Princely India', in *Rearguard Action: Selected Essays in Late Colonial Indian History*, (New Delhi: Sterling Publishers Pvt. Ltd., 1996), p. 177.

18. Arthur Swinson, *The North-West Frontier: People & Events, 1839–1947*, (London: Hutchinson & Co., 1967), p. 258.

19. Curzon to Hamilton, 15 August 1900, Curzon Papers, Mss Eur F111/200.

20. Hamilton to Curzon, 05 September 1900, Curzon Papers, Mss Eur F111/159.

21. See Chapter 2.

22. Curzon to Hamilton, 22 May 1901, Curzon Papers, Mss Eur F111/202.

23. Memorandum on the scheme for the Administration of the NWFP by the Lieutenant Governor of the Punjab, 15 July 1901, Curzon Papers, Mss Eur F111/321.

24. Mackworth Young to Curzon, 20 September 1900, Curzon Papers, Mss Eur F111/202.

25. Young to Curzon, 26 September 1900, Curzon Papers, Mss Eur F111/202.

26. Curzon to Mackworth Young, 23 September 1900, Curzon Papers, Mss Eur F111/202.

27. Curzon to Mackworth Young, 30 September 1900, Curzon Papers, Mss Eur F111/202.

28. Lawrence, *The India We Served*, 160–1.

29. Raleigh to Lawrence, 22 September 1901, Curzon Papers, Mss Eur F111/230.

30. Memorandum . . . by the Lieutenant Governor, 15 July 1901, Curzon Papers, Mss Eur F111/321, p. 1.

31. Capt. G.O. Roos-Keppel, Political Officer, Khyber, 05 May 1901, Memorandum to H.S. Barnes, p. 2, Curzon Papers, Mss Eur F111/322.

32. Khalid bin Sayeed, *Pakistan: The Formative Phase, 1857–1948*, (Karachi: Oxford University Press, 1967), pp. 281–3.

33. Memorandum . . . by the Lieutenant Governor, 15 July 1901, Curzon Papers, Mss Eur F111/321, p. 2.

34. Minutes and Memoranda by the Viceroy and others on Frontier administration, 1899–1904, Curzon Papers, Mss Eur F111/322, p. 8. The statement itself was more or less true, and removal of such places to central control was not new—the exercise had been carried out when the Bombay Government had had Baroda taken away from their command in 1875.

35. Minutes and Memoranda by the Viceroy and Others on Frontier Administration, 1899–1904, Mss Eur F111/322, p. 7.

36. Memorandum . . . by the Lieutenant Governor, 15 July 1901, Curzon Papers, Mss Eur F111/321, p. 4.

37. Curzon to Hamilton, 08 May 1901, Curzon Papers, Mss Eur F111/202.

38. Mackworth Young to Lawrence, 24 July 1901, Curzon Papers, Mss Eur F111/204.

39. Sir Antony Patrick MacDonnell, Indian Civil Service, Governor of UP 1895–1901, Council of India 1903–05.

40. Scott B. Cook, 'The Irish Raj: Social Origins and Careers of Irishmen in the Indian Civil Service, 1855–1914', *Journal of Social History*, 20:3 (Spring, 1987), p. 519.

41. Curzon to Hamilton, 11 April 1900, Curzon Papers, Mss Eur F 111/159.

42. Curzon to Hamilton, 23 April 1900, Curzon Papers, Mss Eur F111/159.

43. Hamilton to Curzon, 16 June 1899, Curzon Papers, Mss Eur F111/158.

44. Curzon to Hamilton, 28 June 1899, Curzon Papers, Mss Eur F111/158.

45. MacDonnell to Curzon, 18 May1900, Curzon Papers, Mss Eur F111/201.

46. Curzon to MacDonnell, 01 June 1900, Curzon Papers, Mss Eur F111/201.

47. Curzon to Hamilton, 12 September 1900, Curzon Papers, Mss Eur F111/159.

48. Curzon to Hamilton, 23 May 1900, Curzon Papers, Mss Eur F111/159.

49. The basic recommendation of the Famine Commission was that relief should not be indiscriminately flung at the people at the slightest sign of scarcity, and that people should be made to work constructively for a minimum wage which would earn them their keep. To this end, it also recommended localised relief works that would have long-lasting regional benefits, as opposed to massive earth-moving camps which would be forgotten after the need for relief passed. For a synopsis, see T.W. Holderness, 'Proceedings of the Government of India in the Dept of Revenue and Agriculture', No. 11, 294, 20th December 1900, MacDonnell Papers, Ms. Eng His. C. 356.

50. R.A.L. Moore to MacDonnell, Indian Famine Commission 1901 Appendix, Vol.1: Evidence of Witnesses, Bombay Presidency. (Calcutta: Office of the Superintendent of Government Printing, 1901), 9, IOR V/26/830/2.

51. MacDonnell to Curzon, 05 August 1901, Curzon Papers, Mss Eur F111/204.

52. Curzon to Hamilton 14 August 1901, Curzon Papers, Mss Eur F111/160.

53. Curzon to MacDonnell, 18 August 1901, Curzon Papers, Mss Eur F111/204.

54. Hamilton to Curzon, 29 August 1901, Curzon Papers, Mss Eur F111/160.

55. For a detailed analysis, see Chapter 3.

56. Curzon to Hamilton, 21 March 1901, Curzon Papers, Mss Eur F111/160.

57. Hamilton to Curzon, 10 April 1901, Curzon Papers, Mss Eur F111/160.

58. Curzon to Hamilton, 16 December 1901, Curzon Papers, Mss Eur F111/160.

59. Bombay Native Newspaper Reports 1903, *Native Opinion*, 26 February 1903, IOR L/R/5/158.

60. Dilks, *Achievement*, p. 80.

61. http://upgovernor.nic.in/harcourtbio.htm, accessed 02 January 2008.

62. Maconochie, *Life in the Indian Civil Service*, p. 126.

63. Catherine Mary Wilson, 'Sir Walter Lawrence and India, 1879–1918', (PhD, Polytechnic of North London, 1991), p. 180.

64. Lawrence, *The India We Served*, 219–20.

65. Sir John Ardagh to Curzon, 07 September 1898, Curzon Papers, Mss Eur F111/220.

66. Lyall to Curzon, 03 May 1901, Curzon Papers, Mss Eur F111/181.

67. A visit to the National Archives of India, New Delhi, in December 2008 to consult the Viceroy's Council's files therein, was abortive as the relevant documents were, according to curatorial staff, 'not traceable'.

68. Memorandum by Sir W. Lee-Warner on the Military Administration in India, 4 May 1905, Kilbracken Papers, Mss Eur F102/61.

69. Lists of Members of the Council of the Governor General from 1859, Curzon Papers, Mss Eur F111/680.

70. Curzon to Ibbetson, 16 September 1903, Curzon Papers, Mss Eur F111/208.

71. Ibbetson to Curzon, 26 March 1904, Curzon Papers, Mss Eur F111/209.

72. Curzon to Dawkins, 24 January 1901, Curzon Papers, Mss Eur F111/181.

73. Curzon to Dawkins, 24 January 1901, Curzon Papers, Mss Eur F111/181.

74. Curzon to Brodrick, 28 October 1903, Midleton Papers, Add. Mss 50074.

75. Curzon to Dawkins, 24 January 1901, Curzon Papers, Mss Eur F111/181.

76. Maconochie, *Life in the Indian Civil Service*, p. 107.

77. Curzon to Brodrick, 12 January 1905, Midleton Papers, Add. Mss 50077.

78. Brodrick to Curzon, 24 February 1905, Curzon Papers, Mss Eur F111/168.

79. Brodrick to Curzon, 30 December 1904, Curzon Papers, Mss Eur F111/168.

80. Curzon to Brodrick, 19 January 1905, Curzon Papers, Mss Eur F111/168.

81. Brodrick to Curzon, 22 December 1904, Curzon Papers, Mss Eur F111/168.

82. Curzon to Brodrick, 01 June 1905, Curzon Papers, Mss Eur F111/168.

5

An Officer and a Gentleman?

ENGLISH HIATUS, AMPTHILL AND THE KITCHENER AFFAIR

This is a principle which I shall always observe in public life. If any subordinate, who disagrees with me, and with whose conduct I have had reason to be seriously dissatisfied, offers me his resignation, either out of pique or bad humour, or a desire to put me in the wrong, I shall not hesitate to accept it.[1]

Curzon to Sir Arthur Godley
14 March 1901

INTRODUCTION

The Kitchener Affair has been exhaustively speculated upon and worked on, however, as a study in backroom intrigue and the importance of the 'political' as also 'intangibles', it has few parallels in the administrative history of the British in India. But studies of Curzon's Viceroyalty invariably relegate it to the trigger cause that ended the Curzon Viceroyalty, rather than an issue in which the political predominated over the administrative or the ethical, not the norm in British India. The only episode of comparable unsavourability was the war time government's dumping of Wavell as Viceroy. As Cohen states, it is also important in that it illustrates, by means of the workings of the Government of India, how an administrative issue pertaining to the internal administration of India became an affair of high significance in determining positions of power in Home and Anglo–Indian politics.[2]

This chapter explores these points, looking closely at the negotiations Kitchener employed to swing opinion against the Viceroy. It also

explores the extent to which the Kitchener affair was used as a
smokescreen by people who would have been only too happy had
Curzon resigned on some other pretext. The chapter also examines
intensively the 'Ampthill angle'—the degree to which Curzon's England
hiatus and Ampthill's acting Viceroyalty enabled Kitchener and the
Home Government to cement a web of intrigue around the Viceroy.
Delegation here proved costly for Curzon; and for Ampthill, sticking up
for Curzon, while being his locum cost him the succession to the
Viceroyalty. To what extent was the India Office used by Kitchener as a
pawn to induce Curzon to resign? What is the reason behind the India
Council's comparative silence on the issue? While some of them publicly
came out in support of Curzon's argument, these protestations do not
seem to have been officially tabled. Nor has their support been logged
by historians, even as it was an astonishing turnaround for a body whose
relationship with the Viceroy had been mutually considered unworkable.
It is especially puzzling because in the case of the Kitchener affair, it
would appear that Curzon was for once in tune with the majoritarian
opinion; that Kitchener should not be allowed to get his way. As the
future governor of the United Provinces wrote,

> K . . . wants some-one [sic] to check him, and if there is friction, as the
> papers say, between him and the Mil Member [sic], I think it is probably an
> argument in favour of a military member. Is friction a bad thing? It seems
> to me to have many advantages. The more experience I get the more
> distrustful I feel (?) of the one-man system. Possibly not being the 'one man'
> affects ones [sic] point of view. [3]

Yet most documentation of the Kitchener Affair, including that of the
seminal King thesis, draws upon the Kitchener/Marker/Salisbury/
Maxwell correspondence, and tends to state what Curzon did, or did
not do, in reaction, and subordinates these points to the argument that
Curzon's piqued offer of resignation was an outcome the India Office
had been angling for. Curzon is presented as a naïve victim; the efforts
within Curzon's team to present their case against Kitchener have not
been utilised; in fact, there is no mention of the fact that he had a

support team. Peter King's, *The Viceroy's Fall: How Kitchener Destroyed Curzon*,[4] is one such; it highlights how Kitchener and the India Office both used each other to oust a Viceroy they both wanted out of India for different reasons. What it leaves out, or at least underplays and does not seek to analyse, is the role of Curzon's subordinates and supporters, especially Lord Ampthill and Curzon's Council, in backing up Curzon's case.

This is in part due to historical evaluation of the Kitchener Affair as being illustrative of Curzon's unworkable relationship with Balfour and Brodrick; their responses to the Curzon—Kitchener struggle are very well documented. The Viceregal team, perhaps to heighten the contrast, has been presented as a one-man entity, an exercise that furthers the image of Curzon as someone lacking in delegation and teamwork skills. But it was not just Curzon who was responsible for handling the Kitchener Affair. The point of first contact for Kitchener was the then Military Member, Sir E. Elles, and it was through him that the matter made its way to Viceregal attention, in terms of its being formally taken up. And, of course, between Kitchener's appointment and Curzon's resignation, the Viceregal chair for eight months was occupied by Curzon's locum, Lord Ampthill, and it was during this time that Kitchener really began a campaign of backstairs intrigue with London. These were three people in very different positions, circumscribed by differing sets of circumstances, and possessing very different temperaments. All this presents a very strong argument for elevating the Kitchener Affair above the level of either a duel between Curzon and the Commander-in-Chief, or presenting it as an example of contemporary Whitehall's cliquey, conspiracy-rife political framework.

At this stage, it becomes necessary to ask why, over the Kitchener affair, Curzon has been highlighted as acting in isolation while Kitchener surrounded himself with a band of his 'boys'? This portrayal is the one constant to be found in the works of the sparring biographers of both. Not only does this present an inaccurate picture of both men's networking skills, especially given that in this matter at least, it was

Curzon who enjoyed vocal and broad-based support from the ICS and Kitchener who operated by means of a loyalist clique; but the contrast seems to be deliberately highlighted just to show exactly how bad it was for Curzon that he did not engage in teamwork. Perhaps Curzon has been portrayed as acting alone because his towering personality easily lends itself to biographic studies, often verging on the hagiographic in the case of his many admirers and contemporaries, of the 'Great Man' school of historiography. Yet neither Curzon nor any other Viceroy in the colonies ever functioned as autonomous kings in their realms. (In any case, the 'lofty colossus' persona has been applied to Kitchener as well; and the single-handed relief of Khartoum sits uneasily with the conniving band of 'boys' who skulked around the C-in-C's Indian lodges.) The Viceroy was not a figurehead; rather, in India he was 'located in an interconnected network of people whose careers were also spent in carving Britain's imperial interests,'[5] incorporating varying levels of authority and power. This portrayal of Curzon acting in isolation may be to show his increasing dislocation from his superiors in London. But when academicians turn to his legislative policy, and his foreign policy, he is portrayed as interacting with his colleagues, even if only to disagree with them as he did with Mackworth Young, so the total omission of any other Indian administrator from analyses of the Kitchener affair is startling. This chapter will therefore devote space to analysing who made up Curzon's team, and how they operated.

Traditionally, analyses of the Kitchener Affair also leave out how Brodrick, Godley, and the India Council did their best to push matters through, partly because historians tend to concentrate on Kitchener and his 'unconstitutional' methods of operation when it came to getting his way and thus ignore the role played by the official persona. Brodrick is not always portrayed as being an active agent; the consensus is that his jealousy of Curzon led him to go along with Kitchener's views, i.e., enabled Kitchener to make him his pawn, but the full extent of his and Godley's duplicity is not always revealed. Thus, the relationship between Kitchener and the India Office over the Military controversy is overlooked, as is the India Office's own stance on the matter. Curzon always complained that Brodrick deliberately obstructed him in London, especially over this issue: but exactly what was it that Brodrick did or did not do? How did he manoeuvre through the sticky affair and come out unscathed even in the eyes of posterity?[6] The point to note here is that Kitchener used the centre of power (the India Office) which properly could have been expected to support Curzon as they were the people responsible for appointing him; Kitchener's constitutional superiors, at the highest level, being the War Office or the Imperial Defence Committee, which Balfour had instituted. The blurring of boundaries between various centres of power was the major contributory factor for the messy intrigue that was the hallmark of the Kitchener Affair.

Cohen's paper presents the Kitchener–Curzon dispute on many levels, as opposed to reducing it to a simplistic analysis of any one façade of the debate. Cohen teases through the strands of authority, perception, and the interpretations of constitutionalisms through means of an open 'European-style' psychoanalytic structure. This chapter moves between a detailed factual narrative and the fluid dynamics of personality assessment to present an integrated account of two overlooked themes in the Kitchener Affair; resignation as an antidote to the most commonly explored theme of clinging on to supreme power- and the role of Lord Ampthill, Acting Viceroy in 1904, again as an antidote to the theme of emphasising the dominance of the dominant and principal actors. The examination of Ampthill's role takes on particular significance as it enables the historian to demonstrate that Curzon too had a team, a support structure and sounding board that functioned as a counterpoint to Kitchener's network of backstairs contacts.

In terms of linkages to the thesis, since the base theme of the thesis is executive power and the checks upon it, this section seeks to examine to what happens when power, or the free exercise of it, is perceived by the individual to have been frustrated. What are the options then open to that individual? One obvious option is resignation. Resignation is important because, apart from obviously emphasising a position of defeat/unsuccessfulness, it can also be used as a position of strength or to show one's immutability on a standpoint. Which of these applied to Curzon in the light of the Kitchener Affair? Resignation is relevant in this context as it is not only an over-riding theme of the Curzon Viceroyalty, but it is about making a standpoint through the voluntary letting go, and non exercising, of power.

The other major contention of the thesis is to examine shared power, or delegated power, and how good was Curzon at it. This section will utilise the Kitchener affair as a medium through which to explore these themes. Moreover, it will examine how shared/delegated power operates and is perceived by those around the individual in office, especially in contrast to 'original' power: in this case the power exercised by Curzon as Viceroy or Kitchener as C-in-C, as opposed to Ampthill taking up the Viceregal chair by default, his status not being that of a 'genuine', but *acting* Viceroy.

It is all the more important to examine this as Curzon was neither comfortable delegating tasks or power to anyone, nor was he comfortable with shared control, precisely because he liked to do everything by himself. This section should also be read in conjunction with Chapter Three, to gain an understanding of how problems in the allocation of power have more to do with the office in question, as opposed to the office holder; as Governor Ampthill did not have Curzon's approbation to the extent he did as acting Viceroy, in part because Curzon was disposed to regard the Madras cadre, and by extension its incumbent head, as disinclined to coordinate with the Centre. In the case of the Viceroyalty though, it being an office he held almost sacred, he was a model of the cooperative senior administrator, perhaps because this was the only way he could ensure a continuation of his legacy in that office.

This section will also look at how power puts individuals in unexpected positions. For example, Ampthill during his early days as Governor of Madras, when the stereotypes attached to the Madras cadre were automatically tacked on to him; but the seniority of that province elevated him to a position where he came closer to being the Viceroy's right-hand man than anyone else in British India.

THEME 1: RESIGNATION

The determining points of Curzon's Viceroyalty all centred on resignation as a theme. George Hamilton resigned in September 1903, which led to St. John Brodrick, with his past love-hate relationship with Curzon, occupying the Secretary of State's chair. Kitchener attempted to resign in September 1904, but his overtly political feint was shot down by Ampthill; nor was Curzon's unenthusiastic offer to resign in October 1904 accepted by Brodrick because it would have seemed inappropriate to accept it. Furthermore, Balfour's concern to keep the Conservatives falling out of power and Brodrick's anxiety to clear his name and prove himself in army affairs after not obligatorily resigning at the War Office,[7] all contributed to Curzon's resignation in 1905.

As an instrument in the exercise of political power, resignation, or the threat of it, was a prominent tactic of the day under Balfour's government: no less than six ministers had resigned in the summer of 1903, and Curzon's made it seven. Resignation tactics gained an especial poignancy because the Conservative government was itself shaky after Salisbury's death till it fell in December 1905, and each resignation had the potential to cause a domino effect, or failing that, to injure the Cabinet in the eyes of Parliament. In fact, much of the Conservative Government's eagerness to resolve the military dispute hinged on the fact that they might be kicked out of office any day, thus making speed crucial and also underscoring the importance of making the scheme impregnable. This determined, very consciously, the specifics of their actions. It was understandable that the Government would choose to stall a resignation such as that of a high-profile soldier like Kitchener's all the more eagerly.

Ampthill, who had turned down Kitchener's resignation in 1904, noted to Curzon in 1905 that he should have let Kitchener resign, as there would then have been no occasion for Curzon to do so.[8] Hence, this section is comprehensively given over to an examination as to why Ampthill did not accept the Commander-in-Chief's resignation; and why, indeed, did the C-in-C see fit to tender his resignation at all. It will also examine the motives behind resignations in contemporary Indian politics: whether it was an expression of helplessness in political affairs and a consequent desire to dissociate oneself from measures one did not approve of but felt to be wrong; or an act of protest that sought to deprive a misguided government of an upstanding civil servant owing to their wrong policies; or finally, because one felt that the measure was indeed insupportable and resigned in a purely altruistic fashion to prove one's point. It will examine the efficacy of resignation as a tool for getting one's point across to the powers that be; as Harcourt Butler noted at the height of the Kitchener controversy, the option of resigning itself signified power over the powerful: 'it must be pleasant to be able to threaten resignation and frighten the powers.'[9]

As Cross and Alderman note, most resignations, or threats thereof, are 'deliberately used to gain political objectives . . . actuated more by pique than policy.'[10] Curzon resigned over a matter of policy; had Kitchener's resignation over the Swan issue been accepted, he could definitively have been said to have resigned over an issue of pique—he had not wanted civilian interference over disciplinary issues in the army. Curzon was much too emotionally involved with India and very sure of the benefit to be accrued to India by having him as Viceroy; and perhaps because of this, felt keenly that it would be better to go than sustain non-expert obstructions to his plans. But it is possible that his many threats to resign went over as attempted blackmail, and 'an over-frequent use of the tactic, particularly over relatively trivial issues [or those that might seem trivial to the other party, as happened with much of Curzon's 'wrongs'], clearly reduces its force, and the minister involved runs the risk of having his bluff called.'[11] As Brodrick commented to Ampthill,

[A]lthough nobody believes he [Curzon] intends to resign . . . if only people . . . could know that the threat of resignation loses force by continual repetition, they would be wary of using that sacred but last 'pièce de résistance' . . . [however] we are most anxious to save his face in any way we can.[12]

In Curzon's case, then, his resignation became a 'striking example of the relative dispensability of the apparently indispensable.'[13]

Interestingly, while Curzon's various threats of resignation, both over the Kitchener affair and other issues are well known, Kitchener himself used the tactic to unsettle the Home Government, and in September 1904 actually resigned, although, as Acting Viceroy, Ampthill did not accept his resignation. This chapter will examine the reasons as to why Ampthill did not accept Kitchener's resignation in the summer of 1904. According to Ampthill himself, as Kitchener had resigned over the issue of penalising a minor captain, he had declined to accept a resignation made on so comparatively petty a matter, probably rightly in terms of political strategy, because 'when a minister does seriously threaten resignation on what is obviously a minor issue it can be seen as evidence that the Government is in a weak position.'[14] Ampthill of course perceived that Kitchener was using the Swan case merely as an excuse to either publicise or force the Supply issue, itself a smokescreen for his campaign of abolishing the post of Military Member.

By mid-1905 Curzon was very much aware of the political angle of the resignation debate—though not that Kitchener was actively using it to his personal advantage. As he noted to Ampthill, 'they [the Cabinet and the Secretary of State] are anxiously considering whether they would lose more by Kitchener's resignation or mine . . . Military prestige is so much greater than Civilian, that the result may be anticipated . . . I am quite ready to go . . .'[15]

But in 1904, Curzon still believed, unlike Ampthill, that he and Kitchener were engaged in an objective struggle to make the Government of India as efficient as possible. It is quite possible that he would have condemned out-of-hand Ampthill's 'self-importance' had he endorsed Kitchener's resignation.

To the last, the Government sought to convince itself that Curzon had not resigned over the affair of the military membership, or that he was using it as an excuse to avoid it being bruited about that the was resigning due to his unpopularity with the Indians because of the Bengal Partition and his inflammatory speech at the Calcutta Convocation of 1904.[16] In fact, the official line supplied to the palace from both Balfour and Brodrick was that Curzon had resigned because he could not cope with the furore the Partition of Bengal had raised.[17]

But Curzon probably resigned from a sense of disillusionment, as did his Military Supply Member, Sir E. Elles, who had handed in his papers in June 1905 as he felt it was time to bring in fresh blood to work the new system and that given the depredations to which he had been subjected, he did not find it any great sacrifice to resign[18]—the latter sentiment one which Curzon had been echoing since 1904.

The point to note is that none of Curzon's supporters resigned in solidarity; something he had confidently predicted they would do. As he said at the time the Dane Treaty was signed in Kabul in 1904, he had not resigned then because,

> my colleagues desired me for a not less momentous affray, namely that raised by the Commander-in-Chief. Here also we are entirely unanimous, and a stronger dispatch never issued from the Government of India. It seems to me inconceivable that the present Government should decide to trample on the Government of India in a matter affecting their own Constitution. Should they do so, I think it not unlikely that the entire Government of India might resign en bloc—a situation which would be without parallel in history . . . If such were the case, I can hardly think that any Viceroy who knew anything of India or its Constitution would agree to take my place. For in the hands of a military autocracy one main sphere of the Government's responsibility would have been cut off and destroyed.[19]

Even Ampthill, who had become one of Curzon's most vocal supporters, did not resign; nor did Barnes on the India Council. Personal career concerns ultimately took precedence over misgivings about the administration of India under what was feared to be on the way to becoming a military autocracy. Elles, it is true, resigned, but then, like Curzon, he was directly affected by the changes. It is not surprising that Curzon never again resigned a political post in his life, because not only did it remove from one the position to influence affairs, it also isolated one politically as nobody politically supported a fallen man. It may be noted here that while Curzon had many supporters who commiserated with him when he resigned, they did not take official steps to overturn any justice they thought might be done him—with the exception of the press-man Lovat Fraser, and later the adventurer Francis Younghusband, and they were not politicians.

Many people resigned when dealing with Kitchener because they could not match his influence at home; hence, it was futile to attempt to reason through his obduracy. As Elles, who tendered his resignation shortly after Curzon's, said,

> Lord Kitchener came out here with a cut-and-dry proposal for abolishing the Military Member and taking the whole administration into his own hands. . . . Personally it would make very little difference to me whether I gave up office in a few months time or completed my five years but . . . it would be a gigantic mistake to place the whole administrative or executive power in the hands of either a powerful Commander-in-Chief or a weak one . . . there is no question of any personal difference between myself and the Commander-in-Chief. We have also always recognised his great prestige and that he had a work to perform out here on behalf of His Majesty's Government. . . . I am very glad to find that Your Excellency thinks my concessions to the Commander-in-Chief reasonable and proper. If he accepts them, I think it should be as a permanent solution of the question, not as an ad interim one.[20]

Yet in spite of that it was them and not Kitchener who suffered in terms of future political advancement. Even those who did were not compelled to resign, for example Ampthill, found their careers stalled as they were seen to have opposed him, in this case not because of Kitchener's direct manoeuvrings, but because the establishment had come to distrust all those who had sided with his 'opponents'. There also seems to have been an impression that Curzon had turned this into a personalised duel between himself and Kitchener and therefore for other officials to take sides (by resigning) in the dispute would be tantamount to partisanship of one statesman/administrator over another. As Arundel wrote to the Law Member,

> [I] have written at some length to the Viceroy entirely and unreservedly confirming the opinion I gave . . . that members of Council should not resign because they differ from the Secy. of S. [*sic*] on an important question of policy. . . . Have begged the Viceroy to set aside his own personal view to resign, out of regard to the public interests at stake and in deference to the united request of his Council and Colleagues.[21]

It would thus appear that the Council, in common with other interpreters of the Kitchener Affair, failed to grasp that Curzon (and Ampthill) did not seek to oppose Kitchener's plans merely because they held them to be affronts to their personal authority, but because they felt the planned reforms would undermine the constitutional paramountcy of civilian over military government in British India. As noted below, Ampthill had experienced some difficulty in persuading his Council to back his stance; it is possible, though unlikely, that they had never been entirely convinced.

The next section examines Ampthill's role in the Kitchener affair and contends that the 'ad interim' status of Ampthill's administration weighed a good deal in deciding what weightage to give to developments in the Kitchener saga while he was in charge of the Viceroyalty. As noted, Elles was concerned that the government might regard any developments as only stopgap arrangements and reopen the matter while Curzon was back in India, whereas Ampthill, initially diffident about his own prowess, did not think the matter should be raised at all till

Curzon resumed office. The section also examines the possibility that Ampthill was emboldened to speak out about his own views on the Kitchener affair, instead of following a line indicated by Curzon or Whitehall, his two masters, precisely because he was an Acting Viceroy. The degree of unusualness (deviation from the standard norm of bureaucratic administration) of the Curzon administration in fact probably freed up a lot of people to express themselves more freely than they might otherwise have done.

THEME 2: AMPTHILL AND THE EXIGENCIES OF EXERCISING DELEGATED POWER: THE LOCUM'S DILEMMA

We will look at Kitchener's campaign in the light of how Ampthill handled it, and also examine issues of timing and how they are pertinent to the high politics of power. This section also examines how the *de jure* status of a governor's tenure in office affected his colleagues. and subordinates interactions with him. It starts off by demonstrating how Ampthill's views developed as he familiarised himself with the Viceregal office, and how these developments—and consequently Ampthill—were regarded in London, with Brodrick (and Kitchener in India) attempting to win over the new Viceroy to Kitchener's point of view. This section also explains how Ampthill reacted to these attempts by London to impose their power over the Government of India by capitalising upon the temporary nature of his office, and how he reacted (and resisted) to this by bringing his own powers of perception to bear on his assessment and dealings with those individuals involved in the Government of India.

Arthur Oliver Villiers Russell, Second Baron Ampthill, Governor of Madras before he was translated to the Acting Viceroyalty at thirty-four, being the youngest man ever to occupy this position,[22] was responsible for handling the most significant incidents that occurred during the Curzon Viceroyalty; the Dane Mission to Kabul and the Younghusband Expedition to Lhasa. The point here is that his was far from an idyllic interlude; in the face of growing uncertainty as to whether Curzon would resume duties for a second term, Ampthill managed to keep the increasingly restive Kitchener at bay for seven months. In fact, Ampthill's handling of the Kitchener affair, with his unwavering emphasis on keeping interference from London out, served better to contain Kitchener than his chief's methods. As has been demonstrated below, Kitchener's camp thought Ampthill's Viceroyalty a fertile preparatory ground for their campaign; but, in fact, the campaign was successfully stalled by the acting Viceroy to a greater degree than has been avowed— in fact, no analyst of the Kitchener Affair has factored in Ampthill's term and contribution, evidence of a gap in historiography and an underestimation of the 'acting' Viceroyalty. 'Acting' does not imply that Ampthill's duties were any lighter merely because he was not a long-term Viceroy; yet the 'ad interim' status of his charge looms large in all correspondence about the governance of India.

The interesting thing is that, as Ampthill's biographer notes, in the run-up to Ampthill's taking over the Viceroyalty, neither Curzon nor Brodrick mentioned the three affairs of paramount importance that Ampthill was to steer the Empire through Tibet, Afghanistan and Kitchener. The private correspondence, ostensibly of such value that it was instrumental in the governing of India, limits itself to details of household arrangements; Curzon reserved the Kitchener topic for when Ampthill came to stay with him a week prior to taking over. So Ampthill was, after all, well-acquainted with the nuances of the question.

From the outset, Ampthill was apprehensive not about the specifics of the question itself (which, like Curzon, he considered unworthy even of debate), but the quarrels discussion of the question could lead to. For this reason he was anxious to settle the question once and for all with as much speed as possible. As he wrote to Brodrick,

> There is another matter in which Lord Kitchener is pressing me very hard and concerning which Lord Curzon can tell you a great deal. He desires that the administrative[23] control of the Supply and Transport Department should

be transferred to the Commander-in-Chief. My colleagues appear to regard it as a comparatively simple and unimportant matter . . . but after a careful study . . . I take it [as] an axiomatic principle that the Executive and Administrative should be sharply divided in Army affairs. Lord Kitchener's proposal is in effect to revert to the system of combining executive and administrative functions under one head, a system which no longer exists in any other army in the world . . . I can see no reason for making even one step in this retrograde direction and I consider that a large question of this kind should not be raised during an 'ad interim' administration . . . it remains to be seen whether my colleagues will . . . rally to my support . . . I have urged Lord Kitchener to accept a compromise suggested by Sir Edmond [sic] Elles . . . strengthening the executive powers . . . he already possesses. If he accepts the suggestion we shall avoid a very difficult and thorny question . . . if not we shall have to fight out the battle in Council and I fear that this latter contingency is the most probable as Lord Kitchener is desperately keen on the subject. He refers to it on every possible and impossible occasion and he even dragged it in the other day on some papers relating to the diseases of camels. I only hope that it will not lead to any serious disagreement between Lord Kitchener and myself.[24]

But Curzon's team, primarily Ampthill at the time concerned, were more concerned with reiterating their case over and over again, to emphasise their constitutional righteousness, as opposed to taking steps to make the British Government see that their case was right, in terms of publicity as well as military angles. As Winston Churchill famously noted about Curzon, he 'thought too much about stating his case and too little about getting things done.'[25] By concentrating upon the advantages of the contemporary system, Curzon's team failed to address, using practical scenarios, the potential flaws in the workability of Kitchener's scheme, flaws that led to Kut. In fact, they explicitly ruled out involving themselves in the military side of the debate; as Ampthill noted when Kitchener tried to explain that he considered the question very important from a military point of view, he did not

pretend to be a judge of the technical military aspect of the case; I can only go on the broad grounds of well-known principle, administrative necessity and public expediency and there I had no hesitation in forming the opinions which I expressed. I greatly regret that a question should have arisen in my time on which there will be a sharp divergence of opinion in Council and particularly one in which I cannot cooperate heartily with you. You say that you have written 'rather strongly'; I hope not in such a way as to import a personal element into the question. We must argue it out on its merits alone.[26]

This was idealistic thinking, very much against the grain of contemporary political life, wherein 'the process of determining . . . policies is . . . a power struggle between individual and departmental views, and much depends on the force a minister can develop in the inter-ministerial contest.'[27] This chapter therefore looks at how Curzon's side engineered, or tried to engineer 1904.

Curzon grumbled continually about the un-workability and unconstitutionality of Kitchener's suggestions, but failed to highlight their potential for causing discord. Another significant comment of note is Ampthill's free admission that he has not carried his Council with him; Curzon often stated this in lesser crises to demonstrate that the Government of India was not a one-man show, but in Ampthill's case, it could only have led the Cabinet to assume he was on the wrong track, possibly influenced by Curzon. Thus a development which, if announced by the Viceroy, would have irrefutably demonstrated his resolve to encourage the idiosyncrasies of individual administrators, only served to further the impression that his locum, possibly indoctrinated by him, was unable to impress his views upon a (rightly) recalcitrant Council.

But it can be seen from the above that Ampthill viewed this as a purely internal matter for the Government of India, and never expected it to spread to London. This might explain why he protested so strongly when he found that it had indeed done so. Indeed, Ampthill, even more than Curzon, very categorically disliked irregular interference from London. In a letter to Curzon he deplored Balfour's 'love of theorizing [sic] on military matters,'[28] and his disinclination to take advice from any but the Imperial Defence Committee he had instituted. Ampthill and Curzon theorized that this was because Balfour and Brodrick were fascinated with the subject of Imperial defence.[29] But the real reason was that Balfour and Brodrick received their input from Kitchener, who, of course, was at the centre of things, and from English sources, and had planted his moles in the Imperial Defence Committee. As Curzon noted about the Imperial Defence Committee, 'I do not know that they know anything . . . about India, and I do the talking, while they ask questions . . .'[30] It was the man-on-the-spot principle at work again.

Ampthill had to contend with two masters when negotiating with Kitchener; Brodrick as Secretary of State, and Curzon, to whom he was answerable; after all he had been parachuted into the Viceroyalty just to facilitate Curzon's assumption of a second terms of office. He also had to contend with the initial intractability of his Council, as well as the problem in itself of how to handle Kitchener and his conduct towards the Military Supply Department. By July he had managed to swing his Council round to his point of view; 'I am very glad,' he wrote to the Law Member, Sir. H. Erle Richards, 'to hear that you are against Lord Kitchener's proposal and that then is a majority of that opinion.'[31]

Kitchener also made efforts to win over Ampthill initially, going down for a weekend at Madras shortly before Ampthill was due to take over as Viceroy. Ampthill reports him to Curzon as being 'most genial and pleasant.' He was in fact encouraged to hope that Kitchener and himself would get along well at Simla.[32] It is also possible that Kitchener was not just trying to disarm Ampthill, but genuinely win him over to his side, especially as it was well known that he had a frictional relationship with Curzon in the early years of his Governorship. A Viceroy who genuinely liked him would prove more conducive to pushing his schemes through.

Ampthill in fact admired the way Curzon handled the Kitchener affair, and thus, if Kitchener, or indeed Balfour and Brodrick, thought it would be easier to push their views through during Curzon's leave, they were mistaken. Ampthill, genuinely flattered at having been asked to step in as Viceroy, was disposed to follow Curzon's line as closely as he could.

> What I admire most is the way in which, while disagreeing with Lord Kitchener, you have shown the greatest possible deference for his views and brought out into strong relief the extraordinary liberty of action which he has thus far enjoyed . . . [but] his is a mind which is not open to argument whether the discussion is based on abstract principles or practical matters of fact.[33]

Kitchener began by going on the attack, endeavouring to show Ampthill that he had the support of the military establishment as a whole.

'My views, as also those of my generals, senior officials of the Supply and Transport Services, are so divergent from his [Elles'] that I think the only way is to take the matter up in Council'—the very thing both Ampthill and Curzon wanted to avoid. He further continued that, 'with the present system I would not willingly accept the responsibility of command in a serious war. In these circumstances if the changes I advocate are not entertained I think you will agree that my position here becomes a false one . . . in the face of the position he [Elles] has taken up I have had to write rather strongly . . . to bring home to the Civilian Members of Council'—thus making it very clear he despised the Council and the fact that as non military personnel they should possess the right to sit in judgement on his plans—'the great importance of the decision to be taken on a highly technical military question.'[34]

At this stage, in fact, Ampthill probably harboured a greater degree of apprehension over the expected showdown with his Council (who, as he had written to Godley, did not share his and Curzon's views about Kitchener's proposed reforms) than of what Kitchener might do by way of political intrigue. He writes to Elles that a note written by him should help dispel many apprehensions the Councillors had held;[35] evidently the Council needed reassurance from an experienced India hand, as they looked upon Ampthill as too young and inexperienced. It is doubtful, however, whether Kitchener or his staff spotted Ampthill's prowess of

perception; they did not like Ampthill and tried to make him out to be
a poor weak creature, further emasculated by the constraints of being a
very young locum to a very autocratic Viceroy. Certainly they were sure
of their infallibility in power as long as Ampthill held the reins, for the
reasons cited above, but they not perceive that Ampthill himself was
aware of the inherent 'political' tinge of the whole affair, preferring
instead to believe that Kitchener was indispensable for the maintenance
of law and order in India, as one of the 'boys' remarked, 'Ampthill is
quite dependent on K.'[36] He was, albeit not in the sense construed by
Marker. The Curzon years were some of the most peaceable in India,
and in any case there was no dearth of capable soldiers. But as was
proved with Curzon in the summer of 1905, Ampthill could not have
politically survived an outright clash with Kitchener, because the entire
Conservative Government considered itself dependent on Kitchener's
image with the public, and counted on that to keep them in office.
Kitchener knew this as well, and given Ampthill's subordinate position
in the administrative hierarchy, was spot on when he commented that,
'Curzon knows that I am practically the only one who understands that
he alone is the real obstacle.'[37] This may have been true in terms of
persons opposing the Viceroy's scheme, but it is clear that Ampthill did
everything he, too, could do to oppose the reforms; had he been Viceroy
instead of Curzon, he would have opposed them in the same manner as
Curzon, but it might have been easier for the Home Government to
recall him—certainly easier than recalling a Viceroy regarded as one of
the foremost Asiatic experts of the time—unless that Viceroy himself
chose to resign.

It has often been observed how Curzon was done in because he failed
to take cognisance of Kitchener's under-handedness. This is true, but
what is surprising is that Ampthill more than Curzon spotted Kitchener's
extreme willingness to resort to tactics that were not quite cricket to get
his way in things, and also his fundamental lack of precision. Ampthill
also displayed skills that enabled him to contain Kitchener. He repeatedly
reiterated his observations about Kitchener to both Brodrick and Godley,

telling them variously that Lord Kitchener 'is not above making hay while the sun shines,'[38] 'has imported a personal note into the discussion which I had been at pains to keep out,'[39] and finally that he 'does not seem to understand argument and resorts to mere declamation himself.'[40] Ampthill was thus quick to perceive that it was the personal and not the constitutional that was paramount in the tussle over the Military Member. He was also quick to sense that Kitchener's staff were intriguing on his behalf, and that they constituted a dangerous opponent precisely because they were so firmly convinced of his greatness that they further fuelled his ego. As he noted, 'Lord Kitchener is badly served by his staff who are very inexperienced and quite new to administrative principles. They back up the great man in all his autocratic actions without having any real knowledge or opinions of their own and only confirm him in his self-confidence.'[41]

But Ampthill, again unlike Curzon (who took much longer to come to a similar conclusion), did not naively assume that the India Office was a disinterested party; he also showed himself very acutely aware of the close relationship Kitchener had managed to establish with the India Office at the cost of that office's estimation of the Government of India: 'Brodrick has got a strange idea into his head that I am not working with Lord Kitchener and keeps on asking me whether Lord Kitchener agrees to this or approves of that . . .'[42]

Ampthill was also aware of the degree to which London's increasing involvement in the Kitchener Affair could damage its chances of being brought to an amicable conclusion, exasperatedly asking both Brodrick and Godley to stop discussing it at Home, as it would further inflame matters in India.[43]

Matters *were* inflamed a month later, however, when Kitchener sent in his resignation to Ampthill, as seen above. Unlike Curzon's spontaneous resignation eleven months later, Kitchener's had been long in the planning. In the July of 1904 he commented that, 'I see a possible chance of resigning before long . . .'[44] The chance came when Kitchener's order for initiating disciplinary action against a Captain Swan was overturned by the Indian Government because it was unconstitutional. Kitchener argued that this damaged his authority within the army, and resigned. He had already previously stated that if he was compelled to resign as C-in-C of the Indian Army, he would retire from military life altogether.

Calculating that the real centre of power was London, and perhaps anticipating that Ampthill would not inform London of his move, Kitchener, in a characteristically roundabout way, had Hubert Mullaly inform Balfour that he (Mullaly) had 'received a telegram from Lord Kitchener in which he instructs me to tell you that he has sent in his resignation and telegraphed details to the Secretary of State for War . . . if his resignation is accepted he intends to retire from the army.'[45] And even then he made no bones about the fact that the Captain Swan affair was no more than a smokescreen, telling Balfour that,

> the immediate cause is a case in which his disciplinary powers have been interfered with, but the whole position assumed by the Military Department . . . render it impossible for him to continue under existing conditions. He tells me that he thinks Sir E. Elles or himself will have to go.[46]

Mullaly's wording as to informing Balfour that Kitchener had sent in his resignation to the Secretary of State for War, altogether bypassing the India Office, further underscores the fact that Kitchener wished to make it emphatic that he did not see any part of the Indian Government as his master; he was first a soldier and then a cog in the wheel of Indian administration.

This epithet set out, starkly and chillingly, the consequences to the Government if Kitchener did not have his way over the Military Member tussle. He would not stay on in India if it was not sorted out, and if he resigned, which in itself would be an electoral blow to any Government given his popularity with the public, he would not stay on in the British army; the ballot box aside, Kitchener had proven himself in Africa, and as noted, there were not many generals who could replace him in the army per se, whatever they did in India.

Ampthill was outraged that Kitchener had even handed in his resignation over such a trifle. As he noted in his private diary of 1904,

> 23.9: Letter from Kitchener placing his resignation in my hands for a reason which was paltry and contemptible.

> 25.9: Wrote another long letter to Kitchener pointing out the folly and mischief of his conduct.

> 26.9: Kitchener came at 3 and stayed till 5. It was a trying interview but at the end he withdrew his resignation and I was able to send off a telegram reassuring the Home Government.[47]

It is likely that in this case both men over-estimated the gravity the other attached to his own stance. Kitchener probably made a protracted stance for the theatrics of it; there is no evidence that Kitchener expected Ampthill to take his threat seriously; to the contrary, he did not think Ampthill would dare endorse his resignation. As he had written to Marker in July 1904 about his possible resignation, he had added that, 'I fear it will be blocked as Ampthill would not like my going in his time.'[48] This was true, inasmuch as it would have been a political catastrophe for Ampthill in the event he had accepted Kitchener's resignation. Letting Kitchener resign in the summer of 1904 would have been political suicide for Ampthill. He would of course have been disowned by the London establishment, and it is also not too clear how Curzon would have viewed such a development. In any case, he would definitely have fulminated about Ampthill's rocking the boat while being left in charge. As he poignantly referred to himself, he was the 'junior man' and would have been heavily criticised for being so inflexible as to let so senior a soldier as Kitchener (one moreover highly esteemed by his grey-haired superiors) go. Kitchener could not have been unaware of this. He also knew that the likelihood of being reinstated at some future date would be greater than if he had resigned while under, say, Curzon, and that a resignation made under Ampthill would be more damaging to Ampthill's career than his own. Thus one must conclude that Kitchener only 'resigned' for the political effect he knew it would create in London.

As a matter of fact, for Kitchener, resignation under Ampthill would have been a masterstroke; in his case, it would not have meant 'failure to carry one's point in the current conflict and in all subsequent conflicts.'[49] The popular assumption, both public and political, would have been that if Kitchener had resigned, it was only because Ampthill had been too pig-headed to see his viewpoint, and Curzon had refused to see it because he did not want to acknowledge his superiority. 'Rank clearly adds to the tactical value of a resignation threat,'[50] and all the more so when there are disparities in ranking and public esteem among contemporaries. In Kitchener's case it was exacerbated by his 'external indispensability; [one's] standing in the world outside the Cabinet room,'[51] which here constituted the press, the British public (and to some extent the Indian public) and above all, the Indian Army. Thus, the 'circumstances in which a resignation threat is made clearly affect its impact.'[52]

Why did Ampthill not accept the resignation? Probably not due to the implications to himself this would have resulted in, as described above, as he was a very 'high-minded, conscientious, and extremely hard working public servant.'[53] The main reason seems to have been that he realised that Kitchener was not really attempting to resign over the Swann case. Ampthill of course realised that this was merely a cover for the real reason, (that the proposals for abolition of the Military Member were not being too well received at Simla) and he guessed very astutely what that was, but he also felt that what had precipitated Kitchener into finally tendering his resignation was the discovery that the Viceroy's Council backed the Viceroy and not Kitchener.[54] As shown above, they were initially disposed to support Kitchener's plans, and thought Ampthill was being too pedantic,[55] but changed their minds after Ampthill produced detailed information from Elles to the effect that

Kitchener's system would not work. But the knowledge of Kitchener's resignation did not become public.

> No one . . . knows of it outside our family circle here . . . I don't know if the Viceroy even told Elles. But of course it will leak out in time. Of course K was immensely relieved when he had done it, and I think and hope the effect will be good. It gave the Govt. a shock and may awaken them to the folly of treating K like any ordinary creature . . . I think on the whole K has found this a dull season with Ampthill.[56]

This was probably true; there is no mention of Kitchener's attempted resignation in Ampthill's letters to England—and to some extent the episode did encourage the home government to prioritise Kitchener over any incumbent Viceroy. But the fact that Kitchener found it a 'dull' season with Ampthill does highlight how effectively the Acting Viceroy managed to keep the general at bay during his months of charge. It may have been that Brodrick and Godley were reluctant to push through reforms under a temporary Viceroy who did not hesitate to make his unfavourable views known, because it would have been seen to be a hollow victory, and also because of the trouble Curzon in England then and later when he went back to India, could cause. They had, of course, much to their regret, already committed to an extension for Curzon as Viceroy. Had they pushed the reforms through, and had Ampthill resigned or laid himself open to dismissal through a refusal to cooperate, and Curzon publicly denounced the process from England in Parliament, and a third new Viceroy been appointed, the transparent political overtones of the affair would have emerged, and it is doubtful if the government could have survived this. Therefore the Home Government could not take advantage of Curzon's absence to put Kitchener's plan into action. Therefore, what could have been a position of weakness for Ampthill was turned, in reality, into a strength.

What is of even more interest is why Kitchener waited till Ampthill was in power to take the first steps, as he knew they would be, towards forcing the issue. Timing would appear to have been very important to

Kitchener, possibly because it would not only have determined how his plans would have been received, but also how he would be perceived by the governmental corpus, dependent on who he had negotiated with. Kitchener's action, in fact, appears to have been out of synch with 'the boys' opinions; Repington noted that they had time on their side to strengthen their case while Lady Curzon was ill, because, 'K would in no case act while a mere locum temens was in power in India.'[57] Obviously the boys were mistaken on this one; or they did not guess that a feint made while a locum was in charge would sufficiently alert the Government as to the damage that would be caused by the real thing, and make them work towards preventing it at all costs. Kitchener probably conjectured that Ampthill would be a pushover, or that he would be amenable to the plan itself (possibly due to the traditional friction between Madras and Simla and the consequent possibility that Ampthill might like to assert himself as Viceroy). It is also possible that he was confident about the long-term success of his plan and did not really think that the attitude of any incumbent Viceroy would be a serious barrier.

The boys did not share Kitchener's precise reasons for deeming timing important; they cogitated endlessly as to the best time to swing Kitchener's plans into action. They might have thought it unseemly for 'K' to be seen tussling with a 'mere locum temens' but they did not relish the idea of him taking on Curzon either in what might have very possibly been an unsuccessful battle. Repington felt that,

> as to the question of expediency, whether it is best to bring matters to a crisis while Curzon is Viceroy, or to await his departure, that is a matter for K to decide . . . my opinion . . . [is] that is better to avoid a collision with Curzon. This moribund Government . . . will always depend on Curzon whether he is at home or in India. He rules them.[58]

And again, 'If I were K I would await this appointment [that of Curzon's successor] before acting, as Curzon has rather a strong following and there is no object in arousing unnecessary opposition.'[59] The boys, apparently, were rather less confident of ultimate success than Kitchener—his apparent risk-taking might in fact have spurred them on to idolise him even more than they already did.

It is also possible that Kitchener was genuinely surprised at Curzon's disapproval of his plans. Kitchener knew of course why Curzon had sanctioned, indeed pressed for, his appointment: to reform the Indian Army. This would immediately have suggested to him that the other top generals, the Military Member in particular, were inadequately equipped for the task; why otherwise would the Viceroy have asked for him? The logical extension of this line of thought would be that the Viceroy would give him a free hand, as indeed he had with other administrators he thought highly of, such as A.P. MacDonnell and Francis Younghusband. Thus Kitchener's obduracy when he found that this was not so, springing from what he judged his task to be, as per his temperament, is understandable if not justifiable. And of course, the Government of India's consent was necessary for all his actions (this was before he embarked on his full-fledged campaign of political intrigue)—but he did not see himself as being bound to work in coordination with it. Rather, as Balfour wrote to him about his views on the matter, 'the existing division of attributes between the Commander-in-Chief and the Military Member of the Council is quite indefensible . . . the remedy is with the Indian Government and I am sure you will see that it is applied . . .'[60] The use of the phrase 'Indian Government' to be oblique about one's exact targets was not limited to Balfour; as noted below, Kitchener also took recourse to it. In any case, Kitchener's thinking was that if the Indian Government under its full time chief was not amenable, it had better be rushed when it was possibly rather more vulnerable and susceptible to strong external influences. This may be one explanation for his attempt to force the issue during Ampthill's time in office; perhaps he hoped that the combination of a temporary Viceroy and a supportive India Office might get him his way. Curzon might or might not come back for a second term, but the possibility was that, if presented with a fait accompli on his return, he might wish to focus on the remaining items on his agenda of reform rather than squabble about what would be difficult to have overturned.

It is possible that following this conjecture, Kitchener's campaign was pitched rather more strongly than it would otherwise have been; the Kitchener camp all seem to have over-estimated the degree of control Curzon by then had over the Home Government. Perhaps they did not know of his wrangles with the India Council or Brodrick, or assumed, as others did, that Curzon got on famously with Brodrick because of their longstanding intimacy. It was the conflagration of Curzon's private contretemps over administrative issues with the India Office and Kitchener's campaign (to achieve his own ends) that did him in. These strands never met on their own until Brodrick took it upon himself to make them meet. This is also a pointer to the fact that just as Kitchener used Balfour's love of military strategising and Brodrick's hostility to Curzon to get his own way, so also they used him to stamp their predominance over the Viceroy.

And given the remote possibility that Ampthill might have accepted his feinted resignation in 1904, it would still have been a lot less damaging to Kitchener than being outmanoeuvred by Curzon. Losing a tussle with a senior Conservative politician—for that was what Curzon was—could have scuppered his political ambitions, of which he had a great many. Here is Repington again, writing to Marker if he knew that K had been,

> in touch with the heads of the Liberal Party and that they know, or think they know, that he would chuck soldiery to become S of S [sic]? . . . Would the gain of such a capable administrator compensate for the loss of K as C-in-C [sic] in a great war? If the Govt. were over thrown would K have gained or lost?[61]

This actually disproves Stephen Cohen's claim that Kitchener did not have any ambitions for even greater military power, but merely wanted to make the army efficient; as a matter of fact, given that around fifty per cent of pro-consuls in the mid-nineteenth century were from military backgrounds, Kitchener was acting perfectly in accordance with the textbook model of assuming, first military, and then administrative, charge of a colony.[62] But it also reveals the calculations which induced Kitchener to set the ball rolling while a locum was in office.

BRODRICK, AMPTHILL, AND KITCHENER

Ampthill might have possessed one sort of power during his incumbency of the Viceroyalty, but the sort of power he customarily exercised: that of the Governor of Madras and its attendant ideological affiliations, influenced the India Office's reactions to *his* reactions to Kitchener. It appears to have been assumed by Brodrick and Godley that the best of the traditions of the Madras and Bombay Presidencies—a grudge against the Viceroy at Simla—would manifest itself in Ampthill's handling of the Viceregal office. They appear to have assumed that Ampthill would be unable to leave off identifying with, and acting as per the traditions of, his old post at Madras. Chapter Three explored the extent to which the Governors utilised their privilege of writing direct to the Secretary of State to turn that official against the Viceroy, and concluded that except Havelock, the Governors did not greatly utilise this 'ancient privilege' to personalise their battles against the Government of India. But they were caught up in the cross-fire between Curzon and Whitehall, and their letters were used as ammunition. It was to be expected that, under such circumstances, the provincial governors *would* be somewhat sandwiched and be hard put to maintain a successful balancing act between the Viceroy and the India Office without jeopardising their political careers. It was Ampthill who, as the longest serving Governor under Curzon, and also Acting Viceroy, bore the brunt of the crossfire,[63] and consequently generated more political interest from the India Office.

This interest at first seems to have been limited to gauging the extent of his readiness to be the India Office's pawn; the fact of that readiness seems to have been assumed to be beyond question. What Brodrick and Godley did not calculate was that, ultimately, as colonial governors, the heads of the Bombay and Madras Presidencies were compelled to identify with India, where the interests of their presidencies were concentrated, as opposed to the political nerve-centre in London. They came to share Curzon's frustrations as to the man-of-action-on-the-spot thwarted by scheming mandarins; after the Akalkot case, where the unanimous decision of the Government of India and the Bombay Government was overturned by Hamilton,[64] Sandhurst wrote that he was 'dismayed as well as amazed . . . the feeling, prevalent enough, will immensely gain strength that no matter what the decision of the Government of India, intrigue and India Office backstairs influence will upset their decisions.'[65] Ampthill in fact is the perfect illustration of the subordinate as a supportive sidekick to his superior, and also the hapless victim by association, drawn into the orbit of his superior, and having, by transference, people react to him only insofar as he was related to his superior and tarring him with the same ideological brush they used for Curzon.

But the l'ese majeste' of Balfour and Godley prevented them from perceiving this shift, charted in Chapter Three, of the Governors' attitudes to the Viceroy. The India Office, and Godley in particular, had been approving of the choice of Ampthill as Curzon's replacement, initially because they found him to be the most suitable candidate for the post, and also because, according to the warrant of precedence, no one else could constitutionally occupy the post. But instead of making a concerted attempt to work the administration with the Acting Viceroy (who confessed to feeling apprehensive as to his new responsibilities), the India Office swung into action to try and use Ampthill for making political points against Curzon. The India Office, first and foremost, used their 'convivial relationship' with Ampthill to demonstrate that it was Curzon, and not themselves, at fault for the recent fallout between Simla and London. Neither Godley nor Brodrick exercised restraint or caution in the attempts to being Ampthill over to 'their side'; primarily by providing him avenues to inveigh against Curzon. Scarcely had Ampthill assumed office when letter after letter filled with innuendoes—criticisms that disclaim any critical intent—against Curzon flowed to him from Godley.[66] Godley and Brodrick adopted a twin line of attack; vocally praising Ampthill's administration over Curzon's, and telling him that Curzon, in England and therefore in close proximity to the India Office, was being the reverse of appreciative of Ampthill's running of the Government of India.[67] And knowing Ampthill's devotion to Madras, Brodrick attempted to play upon the much bruited (but by then no longer extant) Madras–Simla friction by telling him that he did not feel that the Government of India had always backed up Ampthill's plans as Madras Governor, and that he (Brodrick) was now in a position to do so, given that he could liaise openly with Ampthill on central as well as Madras issues.[68] But Ampthill, as seen in Chapter Three, was anxious to compartmentalise the Viceroyalty and the Governorship, and did not fall for the bait; nor did he take Brodrick's offer as anything other than an attempt to drag him into the web of political intrigue that enmeshed the British Government of India throughout 1905. Much too transparently, Brodrick tried the very reverse once Ampthill went back to Madras. Ampthill complained that Brodrick 'has really forced me to go on writing about Government of India affairs in spite of my original determination to mind my own business.'[69] His irritation stemmed not only from dislike of political gossip, but also from the fact that Brodrick, obsessed with the Kitchener affair, paid scant attention to Ampthill's detailing of the needs of Madras Presidency, especially in light of his earlier professed concern.

Godley also most openly hinted to Ampthill the avenues possible if he switched allegiances. Writing to Ampthill after his term as Acting Viceroy had to be extended owing to Mary Curzon's illness, Godley penned, 'You say "it is flattering to know that the extension of your term of office does not cause us anxiety." No indeed, the anxiety that we feel is caused quite otherwise.'[70] Perhaps Godley and Brodrick did sincerely believe that 'the current state of affairs [the strained relations between India and the Home Government] was really the result of your predecessor's system of never taking no for an answer.'[71] Brodrick wrote to Hamilton that did not get any information from Curzon about anything, 'except grumbles . . . [his letters] contrast very unfavourably with those of his *locum temens*.'[72] It is also significant that he stated this to an admirer of Curzon's, who had often backed up Ampthill when his abilities had been called into question by Curzon.

Even after Ampthill stopped being Viceroy and went back to the Governorship of Madras, the India Office continued to write to him about matters that were properly the provenance of the Simla–London correspondence. As Ampthill wrote to his mother, he ended up becoming a close confidante of both Curzon and Brodrick, though his sympathies lay with Curzon; as he noted, 'Both Lord Curzon and Mr Brodrick continue to make me their confidante, and I daresay there is nobody who knows more of the inner history of the business than I do.'[73]

Ampthill lost the Viceroyalty following Curzon's resignation because of this determined resistance of the India Office's blandishments; as seen above, from consulting him on administrative matters long after he had left off being Viceroy, to running a smear campaign against Curzon, and to open injunctions as to political benefits of taking 'their' side, Brodrick left no stone unturned in his quest to get Ampthill back his and Kitchener's campaign. By the time Curzon resigned, however, the India Office apparently seems to have resigned itself to Ampthill's supporting Curzon and not themselves: 'the more I see what you write, the less I feel I can convince you. . . . But when one [having] given a decision in fairly stiff terms, finds that it is ungraciously challenged by the party who considers himself defeated . . .'[74] Of course, he was not offered the succession to the Viceroyalty, as the India Office was now patently aware that he was not the anti-Curzonian entity they had tried so hard to discern in him; after India, as *Le Maistre* notes, he never again held high office. Curzon rightly speculated that Ampthill was disadvantaged by having spoken out in his favour: 'you may also have had to suffer from the misfortune of holding the same views [as myself]. For had you been in the opposite camp, I daresay that you instead of Minto would have been my successor.'[75]

But Brodrick could not yet brush off Ampthill; there was the possibility of Curzon returning immediately to England, in which case it would be Ampthill who would take over as Viceroy again till his successor came out, and thus be responsible for making 'all the preliminary arrangements for working the new scheme' and he could very well sabotage it if he was so inclined to. Brodrick was left with no recourse beyond stating that he would be glad if he (Ampthill) would 'clear your mind of any pro-Kitchener or anti-Kitchener bias with regard to our feelings with regard to your own.'[76] Given that the Kitchener affair was one of the most unsavoury triumphs of un-constitutional behaviour, it was ironic that the government could not send out a more amenable Governor as Acting Viceroy because they were all junior to Ampthill as per the Warrant of Precedence. But there was no need for Ampthill to go up to Simla again, because Minto was sent out; he had been ready for the post since the January of 1903.

Brodrick also took advantage of the privacy of the correspondence between the Secretary of State and the Viceroy to tell Balfour, who did not of course read Ampthill's letters to Brodrick, that Ampthill had said that the Government of India lived in dread of Curzon's return and that Curzon was personally hostile to Ampthill.[77] In India Ampthill was fed the same information, but, receiving as he did a regular correspondence from Curzon, probably did not attach much weight to the fabrication, in fact, it probably made it all the more clear to him that he was embroiled in a political row.

But there had been another, more sinister reason for Brodrick wishing to convert Ampthill over to his views about the Military Administration. The Conservative government was shaky, and if it fell, the Secretary of State would have to go too, and be replaced by a Liberal; and Morley, the eventual successor, was at that time known to be anti-Kitchener.[78] A pro-Kitchener Viceroy safely installed in Calcutta would go a long way towards counteracting London's inclinations.

It was not as though Brodrick and Balfour had Kitchener's regard; he
was aware that they were open to manipulation from the opposing camp.
To the last, Kitchener was anxious as to whether he had successfully
pulled off the coup, writing to Marker, 'I should like to know . . .
whether Brodrick has stuck out about Barrow . . . what a liar the man
is . . .'[79] He probably also knew that, were it not for their hostility to
the Viceroy, and the 'cliquey' nature of the Conservative Cabinet, it
would have been much more difficult to push his proposal through. It
opens up another angle as to why he did not pursue the matter more
aggressively while Curzon was on leave; a weak government might very
well have decided to dispense with him if they happened to be well-
disposed to, and inclined to listen to Ampthill, and this was a likely
possibility, as the governors' and Curzon's contretemps with each other
via the Secretary of State were well known.

The biggest mistake both Ampthill and Curzon made was to assume
that Kitchener's animosity was largely directed at Elles by virtue of his
occupying the Military Member's post, and that they themselves were
only side targets. This translated into letters to London complaining
freely about Kitchener's lack of professional conduct with regard to the
military department, and themselves as being caught in the crossfire.
But the impression that it was Elles he was against was one fostered by
Kitchener himself; as he wrote to the Viceroy, 'the Government of India
has undoubtedly accepted and supported my proposals for Army
improvement, but I cannot say that, owing to the dual control in the
Army, the Military Department has not, in my opinion, been responsible
in some respect for delay in their progress.'[80] This not only had the effect
of reinforcing the impression of his apparent loyalty to Curzon, but also
intimated to the Viceroy that he was not satisfied with the reforms thus
far. They fell into the trap of keeping Kitchener informed of their
correspondence with Brodrick, thus not only alerting Kitchener to what
was going on, but also letting him know how Brodrick assessed him in
his letters to them:

I do not know why the Secretary of State telegraphs privately on this matter which is as official as anything well can be. I shall ask him to make the correspondence official later on so that it may be on record after I have removed myself and my papers from these scenes.[81]

The plaintive tone of Kitchener's letters to the Viceroy and Mary did deceive Curzon into thinking that Kitchener was being straightforward; the only time Curzon tasked him about having taken opinions about military reorganisations from senior generals in the Indian Army and forwarding them on to Lord Roberts, without informing the Viceroy (the move in itself was unconstitutional and could potentially create divisions within the Indian Army) he acknowledged the charge while trying to justify it, in detail. By discussing this, the most trivial bit of his campaign in England, Kitchener managed to throw the Viceroy off guard about his greater plans for gaining support from the Cabinet. And in spite of these admittedly Herculean efforts, he was prepared to bide his time till Curzon left India to put his plans into action; as Curzon repeatedly told Hamilton.[82] This feeling was widespread, and may possibly explain why he did not take Ampthill's warnings seriously, and Brodrick consequently did not exercise the caution he would have in his dealings with Ampthill had he thought the latter to be a confidante of Curzon's.

Ampthill handed over power in December 1904. As seen above, he continued to be involved in discussion of the controversy till he left India. Ampthill's colonial career was yet another victim of the Kitchener–Curzon saga, but he did not complain.

This chapter has demonstrated how 'political structures can undergo incremental change as the result of individual interventions.'[83] In conclusion, it may be observed that while Kitchener managed to have his way over army administration in the short run, the scrapping of the system after Kut meant that the Curzonian side of the debate prevailed. This was, however, long after both men had quit India. It does mean that Curzon failed to get his views across to the people ultimately responsible for Indian legislation. He failed because he was not perceived (by Balfour and Brodrick) to have adequate knowledge of the best way of running an army. In addition to having to contend with this perception (and on the face of it, Kitchener was certainly better qualified than Curzon, let alone Ampthill, to expound on military matters), Curzon failed because he lacked the contacts and *savoir-faire* to build a contrary perception of himself as the person best equipped as to knowledge of what was most suitable *in Indian conditions*. For Brodrick, the Kitchener saga (he and Balfour had in fact warned Curzon against having him out) became an excuse to get rid of a Viceroy with whom he had fallen out. As Curzon observed bitterly to Ampthill when informing him that he had sent in his resignation, 'Brodrick has got me out.'[84] It was also a means of containing a political competitor—a Curzon returning in triumph, would, as Mary forecasted, have been a foregone conclusion as the next Conservative prime ministerial candidate. This way, he was out of active politics until 1915. It also meant that he never again resigned a political post.

Notes

1. Curzon to Godley, 14 March 1901, Curzon Papers, Mss Eur F111/160.
2. Stephen P. Cohen, 'Issue, Role and Personality: The Kitchener-Curzon Dispute'. *Comparative Studies in Society and History*, 10:3, (April 1968), p. 337.
3. Harcourt Butler to H. Erle Richards, 28 April 1905, Butler Papers, Mss Eur F116/18.
4. Peter King, *The Viceroy's Fall: How Kitchener Destroyed Curzon*, (London: Sidgwick and Jackson, 1986).
5. Nicola J. Thomas, 'Mary Curzon: "American Queen of India"', in *Colonial Lives Across the British Empire: Imperial Careering in the Long Nineteenth Century*, David Lambert and Allan Lester (eds.), (Cambridge: Cambridge University Press, 2006), p. 307.
6. In the eyes of his contemporaries, that is. Curzon's fall from grace is too well known, and Kitchener's scheme—and consequently his efforts to put it into operation—was discredited in 1916, a few weeks after he drowned at sea.
7. King, *The Viceroy's Fall*, p. 133.
8. Ampthill to Curzon, 17 August 1905, Ampthill Papers, Mss Eur E233/8.
9. Harcourt Butler to H. Erle Richards, 28 April 1905, Butler Papers, Mss Eur F116/18.

10. R.K. Alderman and J.A. Cross, *The Tactics of Resignation: A Study in British Cabinet Government*, (London: Routledge and Kegan Paul, 1967), 18–19.

11. Ibid., p. 24.

12. Brodrick to Ampthill, 30 June 1905, Ampthill Papers, Mss Eur E233/11.

13. Alderman and Cross, *Tactics of Resignation*, p. 17.

14. Alderman and Cross, *Tactics of Resignation*, p. 41.

15. Curzon to Ampthill, 12 May 1905, Curzon Papers, Mss Eur F11/210.

16. Brodrick to Ampthill, 11 August 1905, Ampthill Papers, Mss Eur E233/12.

17. Brodrick to Knollys, 05 August 1905, and Balfour to Edward VII, 8 August 1905, in King, *The Viceroy's Fall*, p. 204.

18. Elles to Curzon, 13 June 1905, Curzon Papers, Mss Eur F111/210.

19. Curzon to Ampthill, 02 April 1905, Curzon Papers, Mss Eur F111/210.

20. Elles to Ampthill, 09 June 1904, Ampthill Papers, Mss Eur E233/12.

21. Arundel to Richards, 26 June 1905, Erle Richards Papers, Mss Eur F122/2.

22. Dalhousie was thirty-eight years old, when he became Governor General in 1848; post-Mutiny, Ampthill's chief Curzon was just short of forty when he assumed the Viceregal chair in 1899.

23. By transferring administrative, as opposed to executive control, of Supply and Transport to himself, Kitchener would effectively call the shots therein, but would not have to deal with the fine details that execution would have called for.

24. Ampthill to Brodrick, 09 June 1904, Ampthill Papers, Mss Eur E233/37.

25. Churchill, *Great Contemporaries*, p. 243.

26. Ampthill to Kitchener, 11 June 1904, Ampthill Papers, Mss Eur E233/12.

27. Alderman and Cross, *The Tactics of Resignation*, pp. 15–16.

28. Ampthill to Curzon, 19 February 1905, Curzon Papers, Mss Eur F111/210.

29. King, *The Viceroy's Fall*, p. 118.

30. Curzon to Ampthill, 26 May 1904, Curzon Papers, Mss Eur F112/413.

31. Ampthill to Richards, 14 July 1904, Erle Richards Papers, Mss Eur F122/2.

32. Ampthill to Curzon, 09 April 1904, Curzon Papers, Mss Eur F111/209.

33. Ampthill to Curzon, 19 February 1905, Curzon Papers, Mss Eur F111/210.

34. Kitchener to Ampthill, 10 June 1904, Ampthill Papers, Mss Eur E233/12.

35. Ampthill to Elles, 24 July 1904, Ampthill Papers, Mss Eur E233/12.

36. Kitchener to Hubert Hamilton, cited in Hubert Hamilton to Raymond Marker, 20 October 1904, in King, *The Viceroy's Fall*, p. 124.

37. Hubert Hamilton to Marker, 22 September 1904, in King, *The Viceroy's Fall*, p. 125.

38. Ampthill to Godley, 09 June 1904, Ampthill Papers, Mss Eur E233/37.

39. Ampthill to Brodrick, 16 June 1904, Ampthill Papers, Mss Eur E233/37.

40. Ampthill to Godley, 16 June 1904, Ampthill Papers, Mss Eur E233/37.

41. Ampthill to Curzon, 30 June 1904, Ampthill Papers, Mss Eur E233/37.

42. Ampthill to Curzon, 05 July 1904, Ampthill Papers, Mss Eur E233/37.

43. Ampthill to Brodrick, 24 August 1904, and to Godley, 25 August 1904, Ampthill Papers, Mss Eur E233/37.

44. Kitchener to Marker, 14 July 1904, in King, *The Viceroy's Fall*, p. 118.

45. Hubert Mullaly to Balfour, 25 September 1904, Balfour Papers, Add. Mss. 49726.

46. Hubert Mullaly to Balfour, 25 September 1904, Balfour Papers, Add. Mss. 49726.

47. Extract, Diary kept by Ampthill in 1904, Russell Family Private Collection, cited in Le Maistre, 'The Second Baron Ampthill's Governorship of Madras and Viceroyalty', p. 157.

48. Kitchener to Marker, 14 July 1904, in King, *The Viceroy's Fall*, p. 118.

49. Alderman and Cross, *Tactics of Resignation*, p. 16.

50. Ibid., p. 23.

51. Ibid., p. 29.

52. Ibid., p. 33.

53. Curzon to Hamilton, 13 January 1903, Curzon Papers, Mss Eur F111/162.

54. Ampthill to Brodrick, telegram, 24 September 1904, Ampthill Papers, Mss Eur E233/43.

55. See, for example, Ampthill to Brodrick, 09 June 1904, Ampthill Papers, Mss Eur E233/37.

56. Hubert Hamilton to Marker, 20 October 1904, in King, *The Viceroy's Fall*, pp. 126–7.

57. Repington to Marker, 11 October 1904, Kitchener-Marker Papers, Add. Mss. 52277B.

58. Repington to Marker, 23 October 1904, Kitchener-Marker Papers, Add. Mss 52277B.

59. Repington to Marker, 11 October 1904, Kitchener-Marker Papers, Add. Mss 52277B.

60. Balfour to Kitchener, 03 December 1903, Balfour Papers, Add. Mss 49726.

61. Repington to Marker, 08 November 1904, Kitchener-Marker Papers, Add. Mss 52277B.

62. See John W. Cell, *British Colonial Administration in the mid-Nineteenth Century: The Policy-Making Process*, (New Haven/London: Yale University Press, 1970), pp. 48–9.

63. The Ampthill–Brodrick–Curzon relationship has been brilliantly, and almost exclusively covered by Ian Le Maistre in his thesis, 'The Second Baron Ampthill's Governorship of Madras and Viceroyalty, December 1900–February 1906', (M.A., University of Manchester, 1977) and I have drawn heavily on his work, as well as having gone along with his interpretation of events, for the most part. The only omission in *Le Maistre* is an analysis of how Godley fitted in; he was extremely close to Brodrick, a severe critic of Curzon's, and yet seems to have been a neutral observer in Ampthill's estimation, which is curious given Ampthill's pro-Curzon

stance in the Kitchener affair. To what extent did Godley play a role in not having Ampthill succeed Curzon?

64. Bombay had deposed the Raja of Akalkot without bothering to inform Simla. Though annoyed, Simla appears to have gone along with this.

65. Sandhurst to Elgin, 20 August 1898, Elgin Papers, Mss Eur F84/73.

66. See, for example, Godley to Ampthill, 19 May 1904, 31 May 1904, 24 June 1904, 8 July 1904, 18 August 1904, Ampthill Papers, Mss Eur E233/37.

67. Godley to Ampthill, 08 September 1904, Ampthill Papers, Mss Eur E233/37.

68. Brodrick to Ampthill, 22 September 1904, Ampthill Papers, Mss Eur E233/37.

69. Ampthill to Godley, 14 June 1905, Kilbracken Papers, Mss Eur F102/39, cited in Le Maistre, 'The Second Baron Ampthill's Governorship of Madras and Viceroyalty', p. 163.

70. Godley to Ampthill, 11 November 1904, Ampthill Papers, Mss Eur E233/37.

71. Brodrick to Ampthill, 24 June 1904, Ampthill Papers, Mss Eur E233/37.

72. Brodrick to George Hamilton, 17 March 1905, Ampthill Papers, Mss Eur E233/11.

73. Ampthill to his mother, the Dowager Lady Russell, 13 September 1905, Russell Family Private Collection, in *Le Maistre*, 'The Second Baron Ampthill's Governorship of Madras and Viceroyalty', p. 165.

74. Brodrick to Ampthill, 03 August 1905, Ampthill Papers, Mss Eur E233/12.

75. Curzon to Ampthill, 21 September 1905, Ampthill Papers, Mss Eur E233/19, cited in Le Maistre, 'The Second Baron Ampthill's Governorship of Madras and Viceroyalty', p. 165.

76. Brodrick to Ampthill, 18 August 1905, Ampthill Papers, Mss Eur E233/12.

77. Brodrick to Balfour, 03 September 1904, cited in Dilks, *Curzon in India, Vol. 2: Frustration*, p. 145.

78. After taking office, however, he changed his mind and became the new system's most dedicated supporter, engaging in enthusiastic witch-hunts with Godley to root out all 'Curzonians' from the administration of India. But this did not prevent him from ultimately vetoing, in 1909, Kitchener to succeed Minto as Viceroy; Curzon's old friend Hardinge went instead.

79. Kitchener to Raymond Marker, 14 August 1905, Kitchener-Marker Papers, Add. Mss. 52276A.

80. Kitchener to Curzon, 23 February 1905, Curzon Papers, Mss Eur F111/210.

81. Ampthill to Kitchener, 09 July 1905, Ampthill Papers, Mss Eur E233/12.

82. Curzon to Hamilton, 23 May 1903, Curzon Papers, Mss Eur F111/162.

83. Philip G. Cerny, 'The Process of Personal Leadership: The Case of de Gaulle'. *International Political Science Review*, 9:2 (1988), p. 131.

84. Curzon to Ampthill, 12 August 1905, Curzon Papers, Mss Eur F111/211.

6

Communalism, Imperialism, and the Dialogue of Inequality: Curzon and the Indian Intelligentsia

Your Excellency is the true sympathiser and well-wisher of India, and 25 crores of its peoples of different creeds and castes who were always treated alike without any exception or speciality for a particular religion. . . .[1]

— *Wafadar*,
September 1905

* * *

If there has ever been a Viceroy, who is non-suspect . . . has shown a complete impartiality, between all religions, including his own, is it not, by common admission, myself? That anybody should accuse me of favouring one religion at the expense of another, would seem almost incredible.[2]

— Curzon to Sir Denzil Ibbetson,
16 September 1903

That Curzon left India after greatly inflaming Indian nationalism is well-documented; what is rather less documented is that he landed in India to the cheers of the Indians, if not of the ICS. As the *Times* so emphatically put it, 'the advent of no Viceroy has awakened loftier hopes than those held regarding Lord Curzon. The cordial welcome extended to him is an expression of dual desires.'[3] This cordial welcome lasted well into the later stages of his term as Viceroy; in 1901, an Indian newspaper, reacting to Curzon's proclamation that the Indian princes were crucial to the governance of India, commented that,

Lord Curzon, though a Christian, seems to have fully realised the soundness of the view of Manu that the customs and hereditary form of government obtaining among a conquered people should be upheld, even though opposed to those of the conquerors. . . .[4]

Approval was not just confined to the press, which might, after all, be driven by political interests; two highly laudatory Indian works made their appearance while Curzon was still in office; one Hindu, one Muslim, within two years of each other. Empirical proof of Curzon's early popularity with Indians, is a work from Calcutta, later the bastion of the anti-Curzon groundswell; K.C. Roy evaluates in précis all of Curzon's 12 point reform programme, and makes the point that Curzon was liked by Indians not only because of his obvious devotion to India, but because he was given the Viceroyalty on merit and not merely because he happened to be a titled peer of the realm.[5]

The other account was produced by a Hyderabadi Muslim, Syed Sirdar Ali Khan, in 1905,[6] to refute the popular perception that Curzon was not in sympathy with the Indians, and to prove that Indians (and Mohammedans specially) were grateful to him. This work also sounds a note of hero-worship, but provides a strong Indian justification of Curzon's oft-criticised (by the ruling British) acts, such as the Delhi Durbar, which Indians were presumed to have been indifferent to. Some people, at least, fell for his spin, and did not consider the Durbar an excess. Its provenance is even more significant as the Hyderabadis were then supposed to be smarting over the loss of the Berars.

This chapter explores the Viceroyalty as it touched on the following points: the Congress in Western India, Indian Muslims, the Partition of Bengal, and the Punjab Land Alienation Act. These will be explored to find out what view Curzon took of India's religio-political landscape, and assess the reactions of Indians to Curzonian polity, insofar as it touched upon their ethnic identities.

As far as the exercise of power was concerned, even more than in the case of the ICS, in a very basic sense, there can be no ambiguity as to whether Curzon exercised any power over the Indians; he was, after all, the head of the ruling administration. He also very pointedly and consciously refused to be influenced by Indian protestations. Does the historian then conclude that Curzon's relations with the Indians were, in fact, characterised by a classical pattern of dominance? Post-colonial theorists would have us believe that in colonial India, 'power simply stood for a series of inequalities between the ruler and the ruled . . . derived from a general relation—that of Dominance and Subordination.'[7] The question to be asked then is, not whether or to what degree Curzon imposed his will upon the Indians, but whether they thought that he was imposing it upon them. It may be said that Curzon did not have any two-way consultations before going through with the Partition of Bengal; but did the majority of Bengalis resent the move? Hypothetically, they might have made a similar decision if invited to a public mandate.

This chapter seeks to explore three facets that illustrated, or more pertinently, have come to illustrate in a post-Independence, post-Partition and postcolonial scenario, Curzon's Viceroyalty in terms of his relations with Indians; communalism as it is always his alleged 'partition' of Bengal that is used as the showpiece event to back up the 'Divide and Rule' theory, imperialism and its contested interpretations, in this case Curzon's paternalistic/despotic benevolence, and the emergent Indian contention that this 'compassionate conservatism' was merely a set of ideas linked together to keep the Indians from self-governance, which obviously resulted in an unequal dialogue when it came to negotiations between the Indians and the British, especially when, as in the case of the Congress, the Indians were not arguing from a traditionalist viewpoint. Thus, Curzon's appreciation of customised societal modes will be assessed in as a determining factor in his relations with different groups in India.

To explore how these concepts were present on the political scene of India in the early twentieth century, this chapter will thus have three sections, the final one of which will examine what actually were Curzon's views, in the light of his actions towards the two facets of Indian society named, which will be discussed below. The other two sections will examine the facets of power which emerge from his dialogue with the Indian National Congress and the Muslims of British India, the central theme being the Partition of Bengal for the latter, and Curzon's reception in the Bombay Presidency in the former. Given the constraints of Imperial administration, equal attention will be paid to Curzon's expression of his legislation as well as the acts themselves. It will also be explored as to why he evoked such differing reactions across different provinces, while the power balance between him and the Indians was essentially similar across the provinces.

The first section of the chapter makes use of the Congress literature in particular, and material from Western India in general to highlight how the 'political masters of twentieth century India' regarded their Viceroy, and this, too, has a super-abundance of English sources. Linguistic constraints confine the sources for this chapter to translations or compendiums in English of primary sources dealing with the Indians. Some of the relevant works that throw light on Anglo–Muslim relations have already been discussed, and they illustrate how some Indian Muslims did think of themselves as having a separate identity over issues which touched their concerns. These above mentioned turn of the century accounts of Curzon as Viceroy also throw pointers as to how India's Muslims felt about his interest or otherwise in them. The second section, evaluates Curzon's relations with the Indian Muslims in Bengal and the Punjab, and explores the extent to which he co-opted favourable Indian opinion to help him win negotiations with his governors.

It is important to justify one's choices for study. For obvious reasons, the Congress is important as it rose to become a barometer of Indian opinion, and at that time, and consisting as it did of a large number of Bombay luminaries, can be assumed to have been influenced by the political climate there prevalent. The setting of Bombay Presidency, as noted, was also politically volatile; it was wracked by famine and political unrest at the time of Curzon's Viceroyalty. Yet Curzon himself seems to have been very warmly welcomed there, in spite of it being the place from which many prominent Congress leaders hailed: 'The more cordial relations between Europeans and Indians in Western India is very remarkable to one who has been long accustomed to the attitude . . . in other parts of India.'[8] Curzon remarked to Sandhurst that Bombay was the only city which could properly raise a cheer. Indeed, as seen in the preceding chapters, it was the Bombay Government which caused more stir in Calcutta as opposed to the Indians.

Indian Muslims, again, are self-evident objects of study because of the 'partition' of Bengal and the resultant charges of communalism thrown at Curzon. Thus, the Muslim reaction to Curzon and 'his' partition of Bengal will be viewed against the backdrop of the larger theme of Curzon's relations with Muslims across India. There are obviously sub-scts within the major fields of focus; for example, it was the Partition of Bengal that is supposed to have re-galvanized a flagging Indian National Congress (INC). How the exercise of Viceregal power indirectly affected another section of the populace—in a way shows the ultimate lack of control the Raj had—or at least lack of simultaneous control over various peoples in India. Since the INC took up the campaign largely after Curzon left India, it is not within the scope of the thesis, but one can examine how Hindu, or secular Bengalis' views about Curzon changed in the light of the territorial redistribution. What was the reaction of the highly political Bengali intelligentsia? This intersection also provides a platform for examining nascent Hindu–Muslim political interactions in the context of British rule.

In a post-imperial world, this final core chapter is fittingly set in India and is important as it acknowledges and de-homogenises the Indian counterpoint to British power in India. As noted in Chapter One, by their reactions to the exercise of power, the Indians did in fact set limitations and boundaries within which that power could safely be exercised.

DIALOGUE OF INEQUALITY: CURZON, THE INDIAN NATIONAL CONGRESS, AND WESTERN INDIA

Curzon appears to have been well-liked in the Bombay Presidency. When he landed in Bombay on 30 December 1898, it was to great applause. Educated Indians seem to have welcomed in particular his reputation for getting things done. *India* observed that,

> Lord Curzon . . . is in many ways the reverse of his predecessor. He has played a far greater part in the politics of his native land; and he has a strength and self-confidence which should save him from sinking into the mere tool of an official clique. Wilfulness rather than weakness will be the origin of the faults of his rule. . . .[9]

This approval was forthcoming in spite of the fact that Curzon poured scorn upon the Congress, a great proportion of whose members came from Bombay and Pune and the surrounding hinterlands, strictly enforced the plague segregation rules (which caused such riots in Cawnpore), grumbled about the Bombay secretariat, and above all, saw his Viceroyalty coincide with the worst ever famine in Western India. On top of that his relations with the premier western Indian prince, the Gaekwar of Baroda, can at best be described as 'stiff'. Why, then, have the adulatory accolades poured in from this presidency as far as contemporary Indians are concerned? One of the most original commentaries on Curzon has come from a Bombay based caricaturist; H.A. Talcherkar's, *Lord Curzon in Indian Caricature*,[10] is a unique work, which brings together a series of cartoons produced in mainly western Indian papers and discusses their contextual meaning, being all the while greatly appreciative of Curzon. The answer may be found in Gordon Johnson's assertion that Indian politicians of the Victorian period, and the Congress in particular, wanted more rule, not less, from the Government of India.[11] Curzon's prompt tackling of administrative lacunae and the problems that the average Indian faced in his/her daily life—access to justice, racial discrimination, famine, would therefore have appealed to them. It is also possible that Curzon was popular in western India on account of his defence and encouragement of Indians there, primarily in securing the release of the Natu brothers. A striking illustration of his popularity at the zenith of his Viceroyalty in 1903 is evinced by the assertion that the masses were greatly distressed by *bazaar* rumours that the Viceroy intended to return to an English parliamentary career immediately following the triumphal Delhi Durbar and were relieved when Curzon announced he had no intention of doing so. According to the author of that report, this substantiated the 'happy relationship subsisting between the great proconsul and the people . . . the mutual regard between ruler and ruled.'[12] This mid-way through the Viceroyalty production offers an opportunity to vindicate the claim that Curzon did indeed get much admiration from Indians. The book deflects controversial situations with humour, and even goes so far as to quote appreciatively from Kipling's, *White Man's Burden*. The papers Talcherkar drew upon were mostly Gujarati and Marathi papers, and the *Hindi Punch*, with an overwhelmingly Hindu readership.

Further evidence from the Indian press substantiates the assertion that Curzon was admired for his work in India, and not just because he represented a welcome change from the apparently apathetic Elgin. The *Rast Goftar* felt that, in view of the contemporary Asian political situation, 'a strong and experienced Viceroy like Lord Curzon would go far to instil confidence in the people in case certain eventualities occur.'[13] In 1903, the *Voice of India* noted that,

> an extension of his term of office would be infinitely preferable to the importation of a fresh student of India affairs. But when the government majority is dwindling in England, there may be unforeseen contingencies which call more loudly for Lord Curzon's services at home.[14]

Mary Curzon was not the only one who thought that Curzon was indispensable to the Conservatives at both home and abroad.

When the two-year extension to his term was finally announced, even the Tilak-controlled *Kesari* approved of it, though it did speculate that Curzon's real reason for extending his term was 'not the completion of the twelve point reform programme but to ensure the stability of British sway in India and to expand its sphere in Asia.'[15] Yet it did not seem to have any objection to this proposed consolidation of Empire, observing a week later that,

> the Indians, under the aegis of British rule, are receiving valuable political training and are to-day [sic] considerably ahead of other Asiatic peoples. The wealth of the country is no doubt being drained away on an enormous scale, but we must not regret this drain in any way but regard it as the price of our national awakening for which we must ever feel grateful to the British Government.[16]

Of course, it is possible that public opinion tended to be unquestioningly loyalist, *because* the government was the source of all power and authority, and there was as yet no real alternative for persons wishing to attain eminence in public life, except through such participation as the Government of India afforded. In January 1899 a reader of *The Times of India* wrote in to castigate the Congress, because,

> in the last sitting of the Congress, the Congress leaders not only welcomed a person who was convicted by the highest judicial court in the Presidency [Bombay Presidency] of so grave an offence as sedition against Government, but actually took his counsel in their deliberations . . . surely sedition and loyalty cannot be together. . . .[17]

Even the Congress' mouthpiece in London, *India*, which Hamilton saw fit to describe as a 'pernicious little rag', noted with approbation the happiness of the Madras Session of the Congress when Curzon telegraphed an acknowledgement of their professions of loyalty.[18]

Prima facie, it is easy to dismiss Congress' approval of Curzon as being the natural apathy of a then largely loyalist party, or rather a party controlled by the loyalist members, but this would be a fallacy. Bombay was not just a presidency absorbed solely in the furthering of mercantile interests; at the twentieth session of the Indian National Congress, Sir P.M. Mehta articulated at length the delegates' disenchantment at being told by Curzon to devote themselves to science and industry and keep out of politics, as that was a pastime 'not befitting to any subject races.' Mehta's argument against benevolent Curzonian paternalism was that it was,

> equally demoralising to the rulers and the ruled. It ignores all the laws of human progress . . . political agitation there will always be. . . . We prefer to . . . deal with them in the free light of open . . . because we have faith in the innate wisdom, beneficence and righteousness of the English people.[19]

In short they wanted governmental patronage and guidance for their political ambitions, which the Government would not give in spite of their professed loyalty. The counter of the senior administrators to this was that the Congress was not representative, based as it was in Bombay, and composed largely of Parsi intellectuals, thus not encompassing the representatives of the Hindu–Muslim heartland of Hindustan, where the colonial presence most strongly engaged with India.

But it would largely appear that popular reaction to Curzon in Western India was appreciative and hopeful, despite the fact that his most formidable opponents—R.C. Dutt and the Gaekwad of Baroda—were from the Bombay Presidency. Western Indians wanted Curzon and other Englishmen to be reassured of their loyalty, but it would appear that Curzon's line of thought was that if they were loyal, they had better just shut up and get on with being loyal. Curzon's reward for loyalty, as borne out by his Coronation Salt Tax concessions, tended to be concrete financial remissions as opposed to political concessions.

All this was, of course, before the plans for the Partition of Bengal were announced and when in the north, Harcourt Butler was expressing the opinion, now universally elevated to the status of historical fact that by opposing the Congress Curzon was in fact galvanizing it. As he wrote to H. Erle Richards, he felt that Curzon took things 'much too seriously . . . Lord Dufferin, Sir A. Colvin, and now Lord Curzon have shown that the only thing that can put life into the Congress party is denunciation by a Viceroy or a L.G. [sic] . . .'[20] For the Congress themselves, if not for the Bombay Presidency at large, this watershed denunciation came in 1905, with the Calcutta Convocation Speech and the Partition of Bengal.

This section has focused heavily on particular strata from the Bombay Presidency, i.e., the educated urban section, because of the future importance these sections of society were to wield. Curzon might have had fractious relations with the princes of Western India, but these princes did not have an influential voice in forming the structure of the new nation forty-two years later, and their dissentience did not lead them to regard Curzon's Viceroyalty, and the reactions it engendered, as a crucial point in their political existence. The next two sections will look at the reactions Curzon inspired in less politically and economically sophisticated sections of Indian society, which were nevertheless to become participants in one of the largest transfers of population in 1947: Bengal and Punjab.

COMMUNALISM, ORIENTALISM, OR EFFICIENT ADMINISTRATION? CURZON AND THE MUSLIMS OF BRITISH INDIA

While the relations between Curzon and the Indian National Congress (INC) can be best described as characterised by contempt on one side (Curzon's) and wistful attempts for approval on the other, those between Curzon and the Muslims are infinitely more complex. Much of his legislation touched upon Muslim concerns, and evoked varying reactions from them, and there was his own attitude towards them, where traditional Tory pro-Mohammedanism mingled with his contempt for all things Indian and a passionate desire to hold the scales even. In fact, this book contends that the Curzon Viceroyalty marked a political watershed for Indian Muslims, because it gave them—and the rest of India—a glimpse of the advantages affirmative and special legislation could accrue for them. He passed two major pieces of legislation: the Partition of Bengal, and the Punjab Land Alienation Act, became instruments of communalism in Indian politics; the first is yet perceived as the apogee of British tactics of 'Divide and Rule'; the latter, while later helping the rise of the agrarian faction in Punjab politics, was

marred at inception by allegations in the Indian press that it was merely
communally biased affirmative action. This section examines how these
altered power balances in the countryside, as a counterpoint to the
differences among the ICS thrown up by the Land Alienation Act. It
also contends that vigorous British rule leveraged change across Indian
society. This section also deals with the claim that Curzon was being
overtly communal in his interactions with Indians.

Largely inspired by post-1947 readings of the Partition of Bengal,
accusations of communalism stick because Curzon has received largely
favourable appraisals from the subcontinent's Muslims, both contemporary and present day. Even as he states that Curzon never partitioned
Bengal except on purely administrative grounds, K.K. Aziz tries to
reclaim Curzon as a Muslim Viceroy, ranking him[21] as the only
competent Viceroy ever, and claiming that to 'believe everything that
the frustrated Hindus said or wrote about him is to judge a man by the
word of his enemies.'[22] He further pays tribute to Curzon, 'when he
stood for the last time on the shores of India . . . alone amid the waters
of Hindu hostility.'[23] Given that Aziz was chairman of Pakistan's national
body for historical research, his account could be understood to be
dictated by post-Independence dynamics, but what inference does the
modern Indian reader draw from more contemporary comments that
Curzon had 'helped' the Muslims of British India? As will be seen below,
Indian Muslims appear to have persuaded themselves that Curzon had
their special interests at heart. An 'Indian Mahomedan, for example,
devoted three chapters to Curzon in his *British India From Queen
Elizabeth to Lord Reading*,[24] in a descriptive account extensively filled
with long passages from the Viceroy's own speeches. Its major
distinguishing characteristic is its praise of Curzon for ignoring the
Congress as it consisted mainly of Bengalis and Marathas, with whom
the author does not expect the British to identify after having come into
close contact with 'Mohammedan gentry . . . of ancient lineage,'[25] and
the rulers of the Princely States, who he states enjoy the support of the
greatest part of India. According to the author, 'perhaps the assurance

of their existence gave Lord Curzon the strength to ignore the gibes and calumnies of the Congress.'[26] There is an unfortunate grain of truth in this, that Curzon did ignore the Congress, and their claims to be the representative voice of India, on the grounds that they were precisely not that, and that he did aim to cultivate the Indian princes, and he did detest the 'Bengali *babu*', but it is preposterous to add up these elements into the kind of pro-Muslim sentiment that the author so obviously wishes to prove.

The next section thus examines, in the light of charges of communalism, why Indian Muslims (though, in contemporary India, it was not solely they who returned favourable assessments of their '*lat sahib*') gave their approbation to the Curzon Viceroyalty, and how this was received by Curzon.

* * *

When the Anjuman-i-Islamia, Punjab, sent Curzon a telegram deploring his resignation and styling themselves as being representative of Punjabi Muslims, he not only did not dispute this claim, but further stated that the society represented the 'best element of the Mohammedan community in Punjab.'[27] He studiously stayed away from expressing any such sentiments towards the INC. It may have been an exemplification of the classical British attitude towards different types of Indians; and as noted, Curzon was very much in conformity with the societal norms of his own time. Possibly Curzon was rather more sympathetic of Muslim pleading, because he viewed it as being rooted in ethnicity not politics; it is significant that during his rebuttal of the claims of the Madras Mahajan Sabha of 'giving expression to the views of the Indian people,' Curzon refers to the 'Indian public' in the main instance as being 'exclusive of Mohammedan'.[28]

Even if one accepts at face value Curzon's contention that he had 'always taken a great interest in the welfare of [this] most important community,'[29] one needs to isolate the factors behind this. In evaluating why

Curzon paid rather more attention to Muslim special pleading, even if he did not ultimately accord it any more sympathy, one needs to examine the roots of the British attitude to Indian Islam. It was not just a matter of identifying with Muslims after finding Muslim mores and values closer to their own than Hindu ones; Robinson states that up to 1909, British policy, which viewed Muslims as an important part of the South Asia political firmament, was such that it was instrumental in enabling the establishment of a separate Muslim identity.[30] And Curzon more than most, would have known about their political importance, given his extensive pre-Viceregal travels across central Asia and Afghanistan. Finally, in Bengal, Muslims tended to lag behind Hindus in white collar professions.[31] In Punjab, maintaining some kind of economic parity was the basis for the Land Alienation Act, and given the relatively under-developed condition of eastern Bengal, giving it special attention would seem justified.

But Curzon's actions may have had their explanation in a rather more contemporary phenomena; Muslim opinion in Curzon's time was not avowedly political, whereas the Congress was a self-styled politically representative body. 'Giving them hope', would, thus, be construed by Curzon as sending out a signal that for Indians to have political aspirations was acceptable. Finally, Sayyid Ahmad Khan's loyalist legacy hung heavy on Indian Muslims, and may have conditioned them to mouth platitudes of their rulers, and Curzon benefited from the continuation of a policy laid down towards his predecessors. He would not, of course, have been averse to demonstrations of submissive loyalty. Thus, extant dynamics between Curzon and the major emergent political factions in India cannot always be assessed using historically stereotypical modes of thought.

As demonstrated, affirmative action was a prominent characteristic of Curzon's administration. In a reply to an address made to him by the Central National Mahomedan Association, the first pan-Indian association and also the first such Muslim association, the Viceroy stated that the object of British aid was, not to create for you exceptional advantages in the struggle for life—for this your own sense of proportion and fairness has never led you to claim—but to remove the drawbacks under which you formerly laboured and to provide for you an open approach to a fair field.[32]

In 1904, the Home Secretary, H.H. Risley, in note to which the Viceroy gave his full approval, supported the decision to abolish competitive examinations for the Provincial Civil Service in Bombay Madras and Bengal on the grounds that the existing system largely benefited only Hindus, whereas the new system would 'leave us free to deal equitably with the claims of the representatives of different races, religions and localities.'[33] In 1901 the Punjab Government set aside 30 per cent of civil service appointments for Muslims. But he did not approve of people themselves putting forward claims to such privileges, squashing the Anjunman-i-Mufid-i-Ahla-i-Islam by stating that grumbling about the 'patronage' shown to Hindus and requesting greater government backing for Muslims was the 'inevitable concomitant of representations from Mahomedan bodies in these countries.'[34]

Yet in spite of this, Muslim reaction to Curzon largely remains favourable, in part because Indian Muslims tended to feel he was 'on their side'. According to K.K. Aziz again,

in India the Muslims were trusted and respected by their imperial rulers. It was a comforting thought that their aspirations were not disregarded and that their loyalty was appreciated. The Anglo–Muslim amity was as mutual as it was deep.[35]

At a rough count, 22.1 per cent of the condolatory telegrams received upon Curzon's resignation as Viceroy are from Muslims writing as Muslims; an astonishing proportion given that most of the other senders are either Indian princes or British officials. This may of course have something to do with *bazaar* (market) rumours that Curzon had resigned over the issue of the Partition of Bengal. In any case the partition may have fired Muslim sympathies; but in addition, many telegrams laud him for his efforts for Muslim education and preserving

Muslim heritage, or the Land Alienation Act. Henry Beveridge might grumble that 'modern Indian Mohammedans do not care for history,'[36] and imply that they were obsessed only with theology, but Indian Muslims appreciated Curzon because of his efforts to preserve Indian monuments, visible reminders of their glorious past. According to a Gaya notable, 'the Mohammedans ever had praises and blessings for His Excellency whenever they heard of the good work which he was doing for the renovations of their ancient monuments and works of historical interest.'[37] It helped of course that Curzon's undertakings were largely centred among the Mughal edifices of northern India.

The next section thus moves on to the event that is seen as the prelude to the Partition of 1947, the Partition of Bengal, 1905, and examines whether Curzon really did try to regulate appropriation of power between two communities to British liking by this measure.

TERRITORIAL REDISTRIBUTION IN BENGAL

Curzon himself appears to have been well received not only by contemporary Muslims, but also by present Pakistani scholarship, largely because of the measure which has ensured he is so detested by modern Indian and postcolonial historians, *viz.*, the Partition of Bengal. He may have stated that he had 'not offered political concessions, because I do not regard it . . . in the interests of India to do so,'[38] but contemporary Muslim opinion, and modern Pakistani scholarship, less understandably, seem to have regarded the Partition of Bengal as nothing short of a benevolent concession to Muslim concerns. As understandably, given that the reaction to the partition threw Muslims on the defensive, the Hindu historian Tara Chand in fact insinuates that Curzon started off the Pakistan Movement by giving concrete shape to a Muslim province.[39] It makes sense for both parties to label Curzon as communal—in the meanwhile, did Curzon really seek to alter the power balance by a territorial redistribution?

The re-drawing of borders was a major administrative strategy in British India, especially under Curzon. During his term in India he pushed through the creation of the NWFP, bought back the Berars from the Nizam of Hyderabad, renamed the North-Western Provinces, and of course 'partitioned Bengal', which was in fact an umbrella term for reallocating territory between four major regions in eastern India: Bengal, Assam, Orissa, and the Chota Nagpur tribal belt. But the Partition of Bengal, or more precisely, the separation of the eastern part of the Bengali-speaking area from Calcutta, was politically significant because it demonstrated the possible advantages that separate politically and territorially autonomous regions could bring to their inhabitants and the bargaining power that would thus be afforded them vis-à-vis the government. The plan for the Partition was not very enthusiastically received in London, nor by the incumbent Lieutenant Governor, Sir John Bourdillon. Thus when the Partition at last took effect on 11 August 1905, just before Curzon's resignation, the *Charu Mihir* of Mymensingh attributed it to Brodrick's desire to appease Curzon after being compelled to thwart him over the Army and Tibet.[40] The *Sanjivani* of Calcutta, which, like the *Charu Mihir*, opposed the Partition, noted that Curzon had specially replaced Bourdillon with Sir A.H.L. Fraser to effect this.[41] This contention was true, but given that Fraser was one of the proponents of the Partition plan as it took shape,[42] it made sense for Curzon to have him on board, rather than risk a repeat of the Mackworth Young episode in the Punjab in 1901, when the NWFP was created.

Muslim sources universally laud Curzon's decision to redraw the boundaries of Bengal, because of the perceived benefits it brought to the east Bengali Muslims. But it is apparent from Curzon's own speeches that initially he was more concerned about reassuring the populace that there would be no adverse political ramifications arising from a readjustment of territory with Assam, rather than communalism arising out of the partition. It was only when it became apparent that the Calcutta-*mofussil* de-coupling was being touted as a communally divisive scheme that he began playing to Muslim sentiments to drum up support for his scheme. It was one instance where he moulded his strategy in response to Indian public opinion, and it backfired horribly upon him.

Curzon's support for separate Muslim identity is most starkly brought out in his 1904 speech to cheering Muslim landowners before the partition of Bengal, which he said endowed Bengali Muslims with 'a unity . . . they had not enjoyed since the days of the Mussulman . . . kings,'[43] i.e., the Mughal emperors. He stated that this 'Muslim unity' was beneficial because it would 'develop local interests and trade to a degree that is impossible so long as you remain, to use your own words, the appange of another administration.'[44] This appeal to eastern Bengali (and therefore largely Muslim) sentiment is even more significant in view of the fact that the 'Other Administration' was the Calcutta based 'babu' dominated administration, a largely Hindu edifice at loggerheads with Curzon. In the same strain, he continued that the Muslim community, being backward in relation to Hindus, required 'every stimulus and encouragement that we can provide.'[45]

Keay notes that this speech, however, was 'presumably a reference to the heavily Persianised courts of the eighteenth-century nawabs; it may not have had much resonance for east Bengal's mainly low caste converts to Islam. On the other hand it was certainly offensive to the mainly Hindu zamindars . . . so well represented among the Anglophone agitators of Calcutta.'[46] This was something that Curzon, too, was aware of.

While undoubtedly aware of Muslim euphoric sentiments, Curzon seems to have used them as a playing card to win more support from greater numbers of Indians for the administratively convenient manoeuvre. Nevertheless, the Partition of Bengal was most impressive in its impact on communal and British–Hindu–Muslim relations. In fact, this 'masterly British move . . . inaugurated a new era of Muslim politics in India.'[47] It probably highlighted the existence of Muslims as a separate political entity, which could be used to draw and re-draw political formations. Referring to the alleged Hindu Bengali parochialism in opposing the partition when it was touted as being of pan-Indian benefit, a Hyderabadi Muslim states that, 'Mahomedans are not likely to estimate a loyalty of this kind very highly.'[48] Thus at one stroke the writer aligns 'Mahomedans', not only with the British government, but also with the rest of supposedly loyalist India. The same writer states that he is 'voicing the feelings of . . . Mahomedans in particular, when . . . we tender [Lord and Lady Curzon] our humble and grateful thanks.'[49]

The fact that Curzon never even thought of separating Bengal by way of giving a fillip to East Bengali Muslims initially may be confirmed by the UP incidences. If he was really interested in taking affirmative action for Indian Muslims, he would never have acquiesced in legislation effectively weakening the use of the Urdu (Arabic) script in its home ground, as this would have dealt a blow even to those Muslims already doing well in the services. Therefore, this strengthens the theory that he played the Mohammedan card only to drum up local support in east Bengal for his scheme to mitigate the risk of mass protests. When he protested in Parliament at the revocation of partition in 1912, it is true that his strongest protests were on the contention that such a reversal would again subject Muslims to merger in a 'great Hindu province', but by this time the communal situation had changed from his time as Viceroy, and also he viewed the reversal as a breach of trust to a people who had been promised certain advantages as a result of it.[50] This was characteristic of his drive for good administration and fairness to all involved. But others put a communal spin on to it from the start; the Home Department's summary of Curzon's administration does seem to note with satisfaction the communal outcomes of the partition of Bengal.[51] Assuming that Curzon's account of the Partition of Bengal was economic in rationale, i.e., he wanted to break the power of the Hindu dominated Calcutta big shots (cf., Calcutta Corporation Act) so, did he want to pull Muslims out of their economic morass? Or can one conclude that all this was merely a nascent form of pan-Islamism and that it was not overtly religious merely because people living in Victorian times and influenced by the enlightenment simply could not openly think of religion as a basis for pronouncing autonomy? The suspicion that in extolling the communal virtues of Partition, Curzon was trying to win Muslim public support is heightened when he lists out all the educational advantages that would be made available to them and the subsequent aggrandisement of their career prospects—perhaps a response to their own cry that they were educationally backward and needed better facilities?

In fact, the communal angle of the Partition does not seem to have occurred to that 'representative' of the Indian people, the Bombay based Indian National Congress. As late as August 1905, what made *India's* front page was the Kitchener saga (in which Kitchener was vociferously condemned and the Viceroy upheld as the defender of the constitutional principle), and the Viceroy's speech at the Calcutta Convocation. Bengal was only mentioned in the middle of July, when *India* reminded its readers that the 1903 session of the Congress had urged that an Executive Council such as that of Bombay and Madras be appointed in Bengal to assist the Governor in the task of administrating the seventy-eight million under his charge. By implication, they believed the official justification of administrative efficiency necessitating the partition of that province.[52] In fact, the word 'partition' made its appearance for the first time on 11 August 1905.[53] Three thousand miles from Calcutta, the *Indian Spectator* commented that it was not possible to gauge the rights or otherwise of the Partition of Bengal at such a distance, and that as far as they could see, both the old and the new provinces would be large enough to be self-contained, and that the redistribution of territory was not skewed towards giving either bloc an unfair advantage.[54] The *Desabhimani* of Guntur, much closer to the affected presidency, while refraining from comment on the partition itself, noted that it was not creditable of the government to turn a deaf ear to the strong protests currently ongoing in Bengal.[55] But it was from the United Provinces that the most vociferous and coldly-reasoned protests against the Partition of Bengal originated. Allahabad's *Indian People* blamed it upon general Tory policy and called Curzon a despot, and first brought out the charge of

'Divide-and-Rule' on 23 July 1905.[56] The *Citizen* followed suit the next day.[57] But it was Lucknow's *Advocate* that mounted what appear, in retrospective, the most rational arguments against the partition. It began by surmising that people were against the partition because Curzon had not heeded their protests and followed it up with a critique of the redistribution of territory as it stood, which was incomprehensible to most Indians.[58]

It must be noted, of course, that for educated Indians, opposition to the Partition of Bengal was in part informed by their outrage over Curzon's infamous Calcutta Convocation speech the year before. A quick glance at most Indian folktales does in fact bear out Curzon's contention—and the general colonial contention—that cupidity is highly prized in the East. The Indian press opposed the Partition of Bengal on the grounds that anything put forward by the man who had made *that* speech could not but be detrimental to the people's interests. Curiously, the Partition of Bengal was also an occasion for the press to lampoon their fellow Indians for being too dispirited in challenging the Viceroy's handling of the Bengalis. Sections of the press had already bemoaned the lack of an active response to the convocation speech, and the initially solely verbal protests against the Partition confirmed their view that they were 'lacking in manliness'. Calcutta's *Sandhya* thundered that,

> One contemporary has even gone so far as to proclaim a war. And what sort of a war—a war of words. . . . When the Viceroy at the Convocation after inviting everybody to be present there indulged in abuse, why did you not on that occasion protest then and there by leaving the meeting hall? . . . Real spirit you do not possess . . . the only thing you do possess is the capacity of pouring forth torrents of words in public meetings. . . .[59]

It is possible to conclude that some of the outrage over the partition was an overspill of the emotions stirred up by Curzon's Calcutta Convocation speech. Yet this speech was not taken into account when assessing Curzon against Kitchener, or his final departure. This is revealing of the complexities that caused Indians to make connections between the various proclamations and acts promulgated by the Viceroy. On the surface of it, there was no reason why *that* speech should have influenced the people's perception of the Partition of Bengal, especially as it did not negatively influence their decision to back Curzon over Kitchener in the simultaneously ongoing power struggle, nor their overall assessment of him when he departed India. The location may have played a part; Curzon's other speech which has been deemed Orientalist, the 1901 speech at what would become the Aligarh Muslim University, where he stated that the tree of knowledge had shifted its habitat from the East to the West,[60] does not seem to have been cited as an adjunct to the campaign opposing the partition. The press in that province lapped up the proconsul's words, calling it an 'address without a single jarring note of disapproval or of discouragement.'[61] Even the infinitely more fiery Bengali press gave it grudging approval,[62] restricting their grumbles to Curzon's apparent lack of such patronage to Hindu institutions of learning,[63] and asking why he expected Indian students to eschew politics when he himself had 'earned distinction in politics while yet a student.'[64] It does demonstrate that people could be selective about which facets of the Viceregal personality they wished to acknowledge and co-opt when forming an assessment of his actions. Part of the paradox of the convocation speech and the partition appears to be that in the first, Curzon outraged educated Indians by appearing to categorise them under the umbrella term 'liars' (their term) and six months later, sought to alienate them from each other. He may be said to have attempted to actively interfere in their sense of community and nationhood. At the convocation speech he made the very implicit distinction between the two types of public opinion that could be said to exist, or at least that he believed to exist, in the debate over the proposed partition. While he never listened to any public opinion, he still thought that,

> It is a bad symptom when there is one public opinion that is vocal and noisy, and another that is subdued and silent. For the former assumes a prerogative that it does not deserve, while the latter does not exert the influence to which

it is entitled. The true criteria of a public opinion that is to have weight are that it should be representative of many interests. . . .[65]

It was thus that Curzon's Viceroyalty crystallised Indian nationalism, and provided the self-confidence the Indians needed to assert their voice once more in the subcontinent, mostly by means of the 1905 Partition of Bengal. For educated Hindus, the class most intellectually outraged by the events of February and August 1905, this meant forging an identity centred on resistance to the British and their legislation. But while the Muslims 'looked upon the Partition as a blessing,'[66] the revocation of Partition in 1911, while denounced as a betrayal of Muslim interests by the Aligarh intellectuals, does not seem to have aroused Muslim ebullition *locally*. This in fact was the point put forth by the Marquess of Crewe in his rebuttal of Curzon's claim that un-doing the partition was a breach of promise to the East Bengal Muslims. [67] The Partition of Bengal might have forged a sense of unity among all Bengalis, and the encouragement to Muslim separatism it offered was felt among non-Bengali Muslims. Certainly, when the Hindu press outside of Calcutta (i.e., in Bombay) contemplated the redrawing of the administrative map with detached indifference, the pan-Indian Muslim press went public about its support for Curzon as well as his schemes.[68]

It is doubtful whether Curzon initially appreciated the social concerns that Indians raised about the Partition. Curzon, going by his speeches addressing the concerns of the Bengalis, seemed to think that the masses were apprehensive about a part of Bengal being attached to the relatively backward province of Assam. Did they state this because associations might not, like the Congress in the case of the Punjab Land Alienation Act, give voice to the apprehensions about the communal angle involved for fear of damaging communal relations, or is it that the communalism angle, and the perceived protest against it, has been reified or invented by post-independence Indian and Pakistani historians, both of whom thus serve their own interests?

It has been suggested that Curzon's final blueprint for the partition was not too well received in London, with both the Secretary of State and the Prince of Wales being opposed to it, and that this, in turn, enabled the anti-partition agitators to gain the ear of the British establishment.[69] If this is the case, it may be deduced that the Partition of Bengal actually served, in the long-term, to leverage Hindu interests.

In conclusion, Curzon can be said to have played upon diverse, opposing Indian sentiments regarding the Partition of Bengal to gather Indian support for a scheme opposed by another, more vocal section of the local populace. As will be seen below, he did something similar when he manoeuvred a complaisant Indian onto the committee appointed to discuss the Punjab Land Alienation Bill. The nature of the protests against the partition undoubtedly influenced the precise nature of his cartographic re-drawings. He was very obviously not interested in shifting the balance of power from one section of Indians to another, but he was interested in concentrating power in the hands of his administration. If this required playing upon regional differences, then so be it. His primary aim in India was to overhaul the administration so that it functioned efficiently and gave the Indians no cause for discontent, and his counting the Muslims as a separate factor was of significance only insofar as he might have to take their differences into account in maintaining British power in India. The cry of Indian nationalists that he encouraged communalism is nonsense, because for that a sense of collective self-identity would have to have been enforced among the Muslims, and this expression of politicised group consciousness was something he disliked very much in Indians so he would hardly have furthered it himself in any group. As a Bengali Muslim acidly commented, 'the assumption of power by either [Hindu or Muslim] is equally against the interests of the British. Consequently, an ebb tide has set in in [sic] British affections for Muslims. On a visit to Mymensingh Lord Curzon used harsh words in reply to a Muslim petition for government jobs,'[70] this being the speech referred to above.

But to what extent would Muslim society have become politicised if the Bengal Partition had not been mooted? As evidenced in the telegrams received by Curzon on his resignation, and as the Viceroy himself was aware, there were numerous small Muslim societies across India. Would they not have at some point coalesced, or would not one have risen to pan-Indian 'representative' status? The other interesting observation is that during Curzon's time, it was the Central National Mohammedan Association, Calcutta, that was the premier Muslim representative body, with branches across India, and appears to have come close to being a pan-Indian presence. However it seems to have died out for lack of patronage. The Partition of Bengal may have provided the immediate impetus for the politicisation of Muslim associations, but given the numerous associations in which Muslims operated as Muslims across India, it cannot be said that the Partition of Bengal, and therefore Curzon, was directly responsible for the formation of a separatist movement. Maybe for Indians Curzon has become a convenient hanging peg to stick up charges of conservatism and *divide et impera* because of his imperialism and dislike of Indian nationalism, plus the Partition of Bengal. He has become the representative of the British identification with, and championship of, Muslims in Hindu eyes. This is exactly what is suggested by I.H. Qureshi; he posits that Curzon was innocent of communally divisive intentions, and that all ulterior motives regarding the Partition of Bengal were attributed to him by 'the Hindus'.[71]

It is curious that Curzon did not consider the possibility of rising Muslim self-identity and nationalism once the political implications of the Partition of Bengal became clear. In Curzon's case, all his three major 'communal pointers', the Partition of Bengal, the creation of the NWFP, the Punjab Land Alienation Bill, things that would prove crucial for West Pakistan's formation, were a direct result of his attempt to improve law and order. But he never seems to have considered the logical outcome of burgeoning Muslim aspirations to a distinct identity. His main worry was that the people of the frontier could be bought over by the Russians to support a Russian attempt on India, not that these people might want to contend for India themselves.

Of course one can easily attribute this to his combined Russophobia and his complacent imperialism, but the fact is he never raised the bogey of an internal rebellion by any part of Indian society. This curious naïveté may partly be ascribed to his not taking any Indian political aspirations seriously, and this inability to recognise emergent Indian political consciousness meant that when it came to garnering Indian support for the Partition, he played what was interpreted as the communal card to popularise his measure.

The Partition of Bengal, thus, was a case where the communal theme overrode administrative convenience in the eyes of all parties debating the legislation. The next section looks at an instance where legislation, fully intended to be affirmative action, was not vociferously denounced as such, when it could have been, and examines why.

THE PUNJAB LAND ALIENATION ACT, 1900: AFFIRMATIVE ACTION COMMUNALISED?

Land revenue had been the major source of sustenance for Indian governments since the Mughal Emperor Akbar (1542–1605), just as cultivation itself was the major source of sustenance for the vast majority of Indians, even before Akbar. Thus it was one area of reform which engaged with the populace at the most basic level. In the Punjab, Curzon in 1900 enabled the passing of the Punjab Land Alienation Act, a move that the Punjab ICS had been advocating for almost three decades that remedied the transfer of land from peasants into the hands of moneylenders to whom they were in debt. On the surface, this was affirmative action at its best, but it also threw up questions about how balances of power could be altered by proposed and actual legislation. Chapter Four has explored the dynamics between Curzon and the Punjab cadre over the passing of the Act; this section concentrates on dynamics between Indian public opinion and the Government of India.

Firstly, the increasing regulation over the transfer of land undoubtedly played a part in the growing assertiveness and bargaining power of the Muslim cultivator, and created communally drawn political schisms. Secondly, as mentioned in Chapter Four, the Act also threw up deep divisions within the ICS over polity, as much of the Punjab cadre had very specific—and differing—views about the exact provisions of the Act. Thirdly, it brought about a schism between Curzon and Mackworth Young, the governor of the Punjab, as Curzon overrode his views, preferring to fall back upon the views of other senior officers from the Punjab cadre. Finally, it revealed Curzon's capacity for legislation that was appreciated by the people, and in tune with their aspirations of what constituted good governance. The mesh of all these relationships showed how balances of power between two individuals interplayed to swing a decision either way.

The Punjab Land Alienation Act is also important because it was one of the few pieces of legislation during Curzon's time in the enactment of which the Viceroy did not have a leading part. Like many others, the principle behind the act had been mooted long before Curzon came to India, but it was Curzon's contemporaries in the Punjab Government who endeavoured to give it shape. Therefore this is important in analysing the Viceroy's ability to weigh up and decide between the arguments of different factions. As a matter of fact Curzon can be said to have brought his over-bearing personality and clout with the Secretary of State to override the objections of the section of the Punjab Government opposed to the Bill. Barrier notes that the passage of the Bill had been delayed thus far because successive Viceroys, and Elgin in particular, were unable to oppose the authoritarian Punjab cadre, which considered itself the best informed to tackle the problems of the province.[72] While Curzon had not spent years in the Punjab, as the instigator of the successful Punjab Colonies Cultivation scheme, he was in a strong position to throw his support behind Charles Rivaz, one of the main proponents of the Bill. He was able to override Hamilton's urging that the Governor of Punjab be consulted before finalising the specifics of legislation by informing Hamilton that he did not care to consult Mackworth Young as he was too quick to take offence. He was also able to ignore the Secretary of State's wishes that he adopt the plan which would apply the new Bill only to a part of the Punjab, and instead chose the all-Punjab plan he had wished to.[73] Further he was able to use his excellent rapport with Hamilton to ensure that the Bill was passed through the Imperial Legislative Council as opposed to the Punjab Legislative Council, where Mackworth Young could potentially delay its passage until changes were made to his satisfaction.[74] Finally, having won over Hamilton, he was able to get Hamilton to have the Bill passed through in record time through the India Council, where Alfred Lyall opposed its pan-Punjab reach.

The land alienation act was the result of collaboration between Sir Denzil Ibbetson and Charles Rivaz, who pushed it through with Curzon's support, the concerned incumbent Governors of the Punjab, Sir Dennis Fitzpatrick and Sir Mackworth Young, both opposing it, Fitzpatrick being more opposed to the form of legislation than legislation itself. A vast body of largely well-balanced literature can be found with regard to the Land Alienation Act. S.S. Thorburn's *Musalmans and Moneylenders in the Punjab*,[75] was and is an influential backing of the rights of the 'impoverished Muslim peasants' of the Western Punjab, but is now also an illustration of the background atmosphere, ICS and otherwise, that may have prompted Curzon to pass the act. A work that deals extensively with the Viceroy's involvement in the Land Alienation Bill is Gerald Barrier's eponymous monograph.[76] A modern study of the communal impact of the Land Alienation Act is to be found in works that study the overall importance of Punjabi politics in the emergence of Pakistan,[77] thus highlighting how many British moves gave an inadvertent edge to 'separatism', but most of them do not highlight the role of the Viceroy, as opposed to studies of the Bengal Partition, or those of the creation of the NWFP, which go to great lengths to emphasise Curzon's role in reviving these plans.

At the basic, most intrinsic level, the Land Alienation Act became a communal flashpoint because the categories it worked within approximated to religious boundaries as well. The peasants were universally Muslim, and the moneylenders 'alienating' their land, urban Hindus. The guiding motive behind the Punjab Land Alienation Act was, in fact, political peasants, especially Muslim peasants, were the chief fodder for the Indian army and must therefore be kept happy.[78] This was also the reason it was enacted in the Punjab (alienations were a pan-Indian fact of life)—it was the major recruiting ground for the army. As far as the British were concerned, backing Muslim political power served a dual purpose; the 'need for a secure political base led [the] government to cultivate support of . . . landlords, for the same reason it sought the support of Muslims.'[79] The motive was not, however, communal, and the Bill was prompted by the debt situation in the Punjab, and not by any communal disaffection arising out of the supposed stranglehold of Hindu moneylenders upon suffering Muslim peasants. (That such measures were not extended to the rest of India was because there were perfectly good settlement systems in place elsewhere, and also because the rest of India did not supply the flower of the British Indian Army). In spite of all this, and the fact that it was a genuine attempt, along with such things as co-operative credit societies and irrigation programmes, to benefit the people of India (or such sections as the British thought needed benefiting), the Punjab Land Alienation Act of 1900 'formed a link in a chain of measures interpreted by the various religious groups as indicating British favouritism.'[80]

Since revenue settlement was one of the major backbones of the Raj, the local structure of these settlements could not but affect local structures of power and ethnology. In the case of the Punjab Land Alienation Act, it resulted in an affirmation of local Punjabi patterns of inter-communal relations, and at the same time, dissociated these communal relations, at an apparent level, from the overt religious schism prevalent in the rest of India, by cloaking it within a political mould.[81] This was because religious identity and the distinguishing effect it had upon people was co-opted into British administration and so became a practical operative force politically[82] (which meant it would be subsumed into politics). Part of the reason the Punjab Land Alienation Act worked to emphasise Muslim identity in the Punjab was because the target beneficiaries of the act, the Muslims, constituted the 'dominant social category with which the British had in large part identified their rule.'[83] The Muslim factor was incidental though unavoidable, but a bonus for the British because it consolidated and integrated the groups to which the British looked for support to extend their rule in India, i.e., the more feudalistic types. Barrier also states that the Act is an illustration of the fact that British legislative and administrative policy shaped the growth of Indian nationalism.[84] It may also be added that it also illustrates how it was the Indian interpretation of much British policy, and most of Curzon's policies, that dictated their effect on communal and Indo–British relations. It is obvious that all these implications were not lost on Indians themselves because while in 1909, Hindus noted the Punjab Land Alienation Act's detrimental effects on themselves;[85] in 1915, on the threshold of the Lucknow Pact, the press denounced the working of the act.[86] But it was not possible to protest; a fallout of the debate over the economic suitability of the Punjab Land Alienation Act resulted in heightened awareness of communal identities. The Muslim press supported the Bill; the Muslims of Karnal held a meeting to 'thank the government for its "thoughtful" legislation'[87] meanwhile, the Indian National Congress, criticising the Bill on the grounds that it was not transfer of land but British taxation that was pushing Punjabi peasants into debt, was forced to withdraw its protest after its Muslim members protested as they found the Bill beneficial to them, and further protest would have alienated these members.[88] *India*, meanwhile, does not seem to have taken too strong a line against the Punjab Land Alienation Act, confining its remarks to a grumble about the fact that its implementation was confined to the Punjab, when there were comparable figures for alienated land in the other provinces. It reserved its strongest protests for the manner of its implementation; that Curzon and Hamilton had effectively colluded over the passing of the Act, bypassing the normal channels of governance. This, according to *India,* was an 'illustration of the system of interference that is no interference and of the hopelessness of appeal in case Indian opinion proves adverse on any important point.'[89]

As always, the Punjab Land Alienation Act too derived its communal importance from the manner in which it was perceived by Indians, perhaps more than from its actual content. *The Tribune* commented that 'people who are not intelligent enough to comprehend the scope of the Bill will surely attribute it to the policy of 'Divide-and-Rule' some years ago when the government began rightly to shower favours on Mahomedans, the attitude of the authorities was misconstrued and there were constant riots and bloodshed between the two communities . . . the Bill if passed is destined to result in incalculable harm.'[90] While *The Tribune* and the *Civil and Military Gazette* appear to have been the first to inveigh against the bill, the *Mahratta,* the *Hindu Patriot,* the *Paisa Akhbar* all opposed the terms of the bill, what they called for was lower revenue assessments generally and the extension of the Permanent Settlement.[91] In Madras, the papers paid it scant attention until it was actually passed, and then mentioned that since conditions in the Punjab were replicated across India, the government had better address the pan-Indian situation in like fashion. Like its counterparts in the Punjab, the *Amritavachani* of Trichinopoly questioned the ability of the *ryots* to raise money to meet the land revenue if they could not resort to the money-lenders[92]—but the Bill never prevented access to moneylenders for the *ryots*. Mysore's *Vrittanta Patrika* also lamented the fact that the government's benevolence would be inutile unless the peasants checked their tendency to extravagance and their like inclination to borrow money 'sometimes without any intention of returning it at all.'[93] The *Amritavachani* suggested a rather more complex and sophisticated solution to the problem of peasant indebtedness:

> the Government should pass a general Act extending to the whole of India by which the people may get loans from the Government on moderate terms. Although it is true that the Government is not rich enough to undertake

this business, still it can easily raise loans from the rich capitalists who may be anxious to invest their capital in Government loans, and these sums may be lent to the *ryots*.[94]

The local press in Punjab did not feel inclined to put forth an alternative to Punjab Land Alienation Act, and was overwhelmingly in support of the Bill, with articles pouring in from all parts of the province. It was one of the most engaging topics throughout 1900, and in the run-up to the passing of the legislation, Rawalpindi's *Chaudhwin Sadi* emerged as one of the strongest supporters of the Bill, being rather disposed to view it as government benevolence bestowed upon the feckless *zamindars*. Lahore's *Rafiq-i-Hind* also supported the Bill, citing it as the only course of legislation which would appease all sections of the populace: there were other ways to counter agricultural indebtedness, for example the setting up of co-operative banks. But such a measure, the paper pointed out, would hurt the moneylenders, while the Punjab Land Alienation Act did not restrict them from carrying on their business per se, only restricted their repossessing land taken as collateral.[95] The *Dost-i-Hind* and the *Victoria Paper* of Sialkot, meanwhile, were rather more censorious, the later urging the Viceroy not to be misled by the *Rafiq-i-Hind*, and to uphold his impartiality by appointing an independent committee to assess public opinion—which in fact Curzon did—and not to make the Bill retrospective (there was talk of this).[96]

The deliberations of the Indian press formed a parallel to the notes circulating around the Punjab secretariat, as the minutiae of the Bill took shape. Delhi's *Curzon Gazette* expressed the view on 23 March 1900 that peasants might now find it difficult to borrow money to pay land revenue, and would have to auction off their lands to fellow small farmers to do so, but it later advanced the view, on 01 June 1900, that the Bill should be passed into law anyway.[97] Contrarily, Lahore's *Akhbar-i-Am* initially had no reservations about the Bill save that it wanted a tighter definition of 'agriculturist' in April 1900, but by August it was denouncing the Bill's supporters as government flatterers, yet paradoxically continuing to state its faith in Curzon's 'impartiality'.[98] It was at this stage that the *Rafiq-i-Hind* called for a widening of the term 'agriculturist.'[99] By the end of September, however, the *Taj-ul-Akhbar* went so far as to state the new legislation would 'end emigration, banish famines and usher in a reign of contentment and prosperity in the province.'[100]

This slow reversal of the initial suspicion that had greeted the bill was also to be found in official echelons, where resistance was being worn down. In early 1900 a Select Committee formed of six Englishmen and one Indian had been formed. Sir Harnam Singh represented Mackworth Young's opposition to the Bill, as Curzon had not seen fit include the governor on the committee, arguing that his opposition would slow the passage of the bill. Singh had been heir to the *gaddi* of Kapurthala before converting to Christianity, and as noted, opposed the Bill, but he did not just represent the Indian counterpoint to British power. He was Mackworth's protégé, and thus a means for the governor to have his say in the bill even when Curzon had contrived to exclude him. Certainly he made valid points of dissent and in July 1900 a Muslim ex-soldier, retired judge and farmer, the Nawab Mohammed Hyat Khan, was added to the committee, and he happened to be pro-Bill,[101] noting that, 'the lawlessness that has generally resulted from expropriation . . . is a grave political danger . . . dacoits have been known to say that [they] only wanted to avenge their wrongs on the moneylenders.'[102] Others went further in elaborating the political danger caused by alienations to non-peasants holders. Even Harnam Singh, though writing for purposes entirely contrary to the Nawab's, opined that the,

> Land Alienation Bill is much resented by money-lenders . . . people were in difficulties and there were not wanting persons to stir them up and to tell them that now was the time to avenge themselves on their tyrants, and so dacoities began . . . committed by Muhammadan *zamindars* . . . and the persons robbed were money-lenders.[103]

It is true that that Punjab Land Alienation Act was a response to the political danger of alienation; this aspect of land economy in fact was a direct result of the dynamics of the Mutiny, in which it was observed that perceived neglect of a religion(s) could spark off revolts, and locally, that the Punjabis stood behind the British.[104]

The Punjab Land Alienation Act was experimental legislation,[105] and extraordinary in view of the previous attitude of laissez-faire adopted by the British in India. Barrier thus argues that only a Viceroy like Curzon, whose preferred mode of governance was paternal—and despotic-benevolence towards the people, could have pushed it through.[106] In fact, the Punjab Land Alienation Act, like most of Curzon's other measures which were designed to that aim, succeeded in binding the authority of the state to the structure of indigenous society itself.[107] As the twentieth century wore on, it became the means of keeping the Punjab loyal.

In hindsight therefore, Curzon's 'interest in the peasantry was suspected; national leaders saw in it a subtle attempt to attach [them] to the British Regime and to withdraw them from Indian political influence.'[108] It was not as though the Act had even originated from the Viceroy; as seen above and in Chapter Four, it was being debated by the ICS for two and a half decades before Curzon came to India. But as Ampthill had once noted, in India all acts were seen as originating in the person of the Viceroy and it was widely believed that he had the powers to modify any piece of legislation if he so chose. Curzon thus far had done nothing to dispel that impression. And so strong was Curzon's reputation as an even-handed Viceroy that in the early stages of the discussion of the bill, the press felt he could not but withdraw it once its deleterious effects upon the peasants were made manifest to him, as also the fact that certain sections of Indians did not approve of the proposed legislation. The *Tribune* made the facile suggestion that,

> Lord Curzon . . . has the great gift of being able to put himself in the position of the governed. If we proceed in the proper manner, lay the pros and cons of the case clearly before him, let it be evident to him that the proposed piece of legislation will do a vast deal more harm than good . . . we are sure the bill . . . will be sufficiently modified to render it innocuous.[109]

This was very much in keeping with the role that the Punjab press appeared to have assigned to Curzon—that of *maa-baap* of the people. This province offered minimal political analysis of Curzon's assumption of office in 1899. For almost a month after he landed in India, the Punjab press had nothing to say about the new Viceroy—or indeed the outgoing one—until Lahore's *Wafadar* expressed the hope that he might do something to alleviate the miserable financial [*sic*] condition of the people.[110]

But Curzon was self-confessedly insensitive to Indian appeals to his 'good nature' and particularly disliked the sort of harping on constitutionalisms that contemporary Indians were wont to employ in the appeals, and over the case of the Punjab Land Alienation Act, he appears to have been strongly convinced by Rivaz to push it through without modification. His stance over the passing of the Punjab Land Alienation Bill demonstrates Curzon's disregard of Indian opinion even when it was not aligned in opposition to his plans. Of course, the inclusion of Sir Harnam Singh, and indeed the constitution of the Select Committee itself, was in deference to critical opinion that Indian public opinion must be taken into account before passing the legislation through, but as seen above, Curzon managed to counter this by putting his own Indians on the committee as well, and in any case the press accorded the Bill its cautious approbation as it passed into law.

Conclusion

In this chapter we have gone against the grain by looking at two sections of Indian society that accorded Curzon a simultaneous mix of approbation and regretful condemnation, as opposed to the universal post-colonial condemnation of him. Thus we can see how perceptions of the figurehead of imperial authority were by no means uniform across India. The second section shows how attempts to redress existing inequalities and hold the balance even between different strata of Indians backfired horribly. This would assume that British interference reset the existing balance of power across the mofussil. As Anil Seal has noted, the power structure of the Raj gave rise to an Indian counterpart that took its character from its engagements with the original.[111] We have also seen how Indians were able to appropriate Curzon's actions to whatever mood suited them.

Reactions to Curzon's resignation, then, were understandably coloured by the very recent Partition of Bengal, especially as it was one measure which was perceived by the Indians as directly affecting them. Bengali papers—at least those that had opposed the partition—expressed a certain amount of rejoicing. The *Amrita Bazar Patrika*, however, noted with sympathy that Curzon 'had been made to suffer a serious humiliation in the eyes of the world,' but also forbore to point out that they saw in this 'the hand of justice for His Excellency's series of repressive acts towards a people who were prepared to honour and love him.'[112]

This did not mean a total repudiation of all that Curzon stood for. When he resigned *India* proclaimed him to be 'a victim of Lord Kitchener's ruthlessness, or to Mr Chamberlain's pushfulness [*sic*], or to both, operating upon the amazing weakness and instability of the Secretary of State for India and the Home Government.'[113] In Madras, public opinion offered yet more unequivocal support, the *Hindu Nesan* using the opportunity to ask how it was possible for Indians to enjoy privileges, when the Governor General himself, responsible for the proper administration of the whole country, was not accorded full powers.[114]

But, ICS opinion tends to the view that ultimately whatever Curzon did in India did not matter in the long run, nor did it greatly affect the country. As hypothesised at the start of this thesis, ultimately Curzon did not have any direct influence upon the development of Indian national consciousness. As Evan Maconochie, Denzil Ibbetson's son-in-law put it, it may be admitted that he set the brains of all communities working with a new vigour and, to that extent, may have given an impetus to certain developments. But the growth of the nationalist sense and of the desire for self-determination is not the work of one man, and he a foreigner, however dominant his personality. . . . He came at a period when the old order was changing, and left India different in outlook and temper to that which he found . . . [but] in the conditions of our Indian Empire the coming of unrest was inevitable. . . .[115]

This thesis has shown how much Curzon tried to do, and get others to do, according to what he judged best, so that unrest, even if inevitable, could not be said to have been provoked by British actions. The next chapter, the final one of the book, examines the barriers to Curzon's exercise of unfettered power in India.

Notes

1. Telegram, 228 Mohammed Fazl-ud-din, editor and proprietor, *Wafadar*, Lahore, 1 September 1905, in Letters and Telegrams received on the occasion of the Resignation of His Excellency Lord Curzon, Viceroy and Governor General of India, Curzon Papers, Mss Eur F 111/420.
2. Curzon to Sir Denzil Ibbetson, 16 September 1903, Private Letter, Curzon Papers, Mss Eur F 111/208.
3. *The Times of India*, 07 January 1899, British Library Newspaper Collection.
4. *Bangavasi*, 27 April 1901, Bengal Native Newspaper Reports, L/R/5/27.
5. Krishna Chandra Roy, *Some Desultory Notes on Lord Curzon's Work in India*.
6. Syed Sirdar Ali Khan, *Lord Curzon's Administration of India: What he Promised, What he Performed*, (Bombay: Times Press, 1905).
7. Ranajit Guha, *Dominance without Hegemony: History and Power in Colonial India*, (Cambridge, Mass.: Harvard University Press, 1997), p. 20.
8. Lionel Ashburner, Bombay Civil Service, quoted in Martineau, *The Life and Correspondence of Sir Bartle Frere*, Vol. 1, p. 29.
9. *India*, 06 January 1899.
10. H.A. Talcherkar, *Lord Curzon in Indian Caricature*, (Bombay: Babajee Sakharam & Co., 1902).
11. Gordon Johnson, *Provincial Politics and Indian Nationalism: Bombay and the Indian National Congress, 1880–1915*, (Cambridge: Cambridge University Press, 1973), p. 14.
12. Talcherkar, *Lord Curzon in Indian Caricature*, p. 45.
13. *Rast Goftar*, 03 May 1903, Bombay Native Newspaper Reports, IOR L/R/5/158.

14. *Voice of India*, 28 February 1903, Bombay Native Newspaper Reports, IOR L/R/5/158.

15. *Kesari*, 11 August 1903, Bombay Native Newspaper Reports, IOR L/R/5/158.

16. *Kesari*, 18 August 1903, Bombay Native Newspaper Reports, IOR L/R/5/158.

17. 'A Hindoo', *The Times of India*, 21 January 1899.

18. *India,* 03 February 1899.

19. Sir P.M. Mehta, speech at the Bombay Session of the INC, cited in Notable Utterances at the National Congress of December 1904 (n.p., n.d.), British Library.

20. Harcourt Butler to H. Erle Richards, 14 February 1905, Butler Papers, Mss Eur F116/18.

21. K.K. Aziz, *The British in India: A Study in Imperialism*, (Islamabad: National Commission on Historical and Cultural Research, 1976), p. 144.

22. Aziz, *The British in India*, p. 80.

23. Ibid., p. 82.

24. An Indian Mahomedan, *British India from Queen Elizabeth to Lord Reading*, (London: Issac Pilman, 1926).

25. An Indian Mahomedan, *British India from Queen Elizabeth to Lord Reading*, p. 451.

26. Ibid., p. 451.

27. Viceroy to Anjuman-i-Islamia, 28 October 1905, Letters and Telegrams received on the occasion of the Resignation of His Excellency, Curzon Papers, Mss Eur F111/420.

28. George Curzon, speech of December 11, 1900, cited in Ronaldshay, *Life of Lord Curzon Vol. 2*, p. 151.

29. Reply, Viceroy to President, National Mohammedan Association, Bombay, 23 August 1905, Curzon Papers, Mss Eur F111/420.

30. Francis Robinson, *Separatism Among Indian Muslims: The Politics of the United Provinces' Muslims, 1860–1923*, (Cambridge: Cambridge University Press, 1974), p. 349.

31. For statistics see Anil Baran Ray, 'Communal Attitudes to British Policy: The Case of the Partition of Bengal 1905', *Social Scientist*, 6:5, (Dec 1977): p. 43.

32. George Curzon, Viceroy to Central National Mahommedan Association, 31 January 1899, in *Speeches by H.E. Lord Curzon of Kedleston, Viceroy and Governor-General of India, Vol 1 1898–1900*, (Calcutta: Office of the Superintendent of Government Printing, 1900), pp. 37–8. [pp. 36–9].

33. H.H. Risley, Minute, 25 April 1904, GIO, Home Education, May 1904, progs 67076A. Cited in Richard P. Cronin, 'British Policy and Administration in Bengal, 1885–1912', in *British Imperial Policy in India and Sri Lanka*, Barrier and Crane (eds.), p. 184.

34. George Curzon, Viceroy to Anjunman-i-Mufid-i-Ahla-i-Islam, 11 December 1900, in *Speeches by H.E. Lord Curzon of Kedleston, Vol 2:1902*, p. 171.

35. K.K. Aziz. *The Making of Pakistan: A Study in Nationalism*, (Karachi: National Book Foundation, 1977), p. 80.

36. Henry Beveridge, 01 February 1900, *Note on the Decay of Persian Mss in India*, Curzon Papers, Mss Eur F112/427.

37. Telegram, Kazi Farzand Ahmed Khan Bahadur, Gaya, 25 August 1905, Letters and Telegrams received on the occasion of the resignation of His Excellency, Curzon Papers, Mss Eur F 111/420.

38. George Curzon, Speech at the Byculla Club, 16 November 1905, in *Lord Curzon in India*, Raleigh (ed.), p. 585.

39. Tara Chand, *History of the Freedom Movement in India, Vol.4*, (New Delhi: Publications Division, Ministry of Information & Broadcasting, Govt. of India, 1972), p. 317.

40. *Charu Mihir*, 11 July 1905, Bengal Native Newspaper Reports, IOR L/R/5/31.

41. *Sanjivani*, 13 July 1905, Bengal Native Newspaper Reports, IOR/L/R/5/31.

42. Katherine Prior, 'Sir Andrew Henderson Leith Fraser', Dictionary of National Biography, available from http://www.oxforddnb.com/view/article/33248?&docPos=72&backToResults=, accessed 13 August 2008.

43. Speech, Curzon, cited in Peter Hardy, *The Muslims of British India*, (Cambridge: Cambridge University Press, 1972), p. 150.

44. George Curzon, 'Addresses at Dacca', in *Speeches by H.E. Lord Curzon of Kedleston, Viceroy and Governor-General of India, Vol. III: 1902–04*, p. 303.

45. George Curzon, 'Laying the Foundation Stone of the New College at Dacca', in *Speeches by H.E. Lord Curzon of Kedleston, Viceroy and Governor-General of India, Vol. III: 1902–04*, p. 308.

46. John Keay, *India: A History*, (London: Harper Perennial, 2004), p. 464.

47. N. Ahmad, *Muslim Separatism in British India: A Retrospective Study*, (Lahore: Ferozsons Ltd., 1991), p. 23.

48. Syed Sirdar Ali Khan, *Lord Curzon's Administration of India*, p. 40.

49. Ibid., p. 119.

50. The Govt. of India: Debate on the Recent Changes, 21 February 1912, Vol. 2, No 4, 150–1, Curzon Papers, Mss Eur F112/592.

51. Summary of Lord Curzon's administration: Home Department, Curzon Papers, Mss Eur F111/518, pp. 66–7.

52. *India*, 14 July 1905.

53. *India*, 11 August 1905.

54. *Indian Spectator*, 29 July 1905, Bombay Native Newspaper Reports, IOR L/R/5/160.

55. *Desabhimani*, 5 August 1905, Madras Native Newspaper Reports, IOR/L/R/5/185.

56. *Indian People*, 23 July 1905, United Provinces Native Newspaper Reports, IOR L/R/5/81.

57. *Citizen*, 24 July 1905, United Provinces Native Newspaper Reports, IOR L/R/5/81.

58. *Advocate*, 13 and 24 July 1905, United Provinces Native Newspaper Reports, IOR L/R/5/81.

59. *Sandhya,* 18 July 1905, Bengal Native Newspaper Reports, IOR L/R/5/31.

60. George Curzon, *Lord Curzon in India*, Sir Thomas Raleigh (ed.), p. 477.

61. *Indian Daily Mail*, 02 May 1901, United Provinces Native Newspaper Reports 1901, L/R/5/78.

62. *Prabhat*, 04 May 1901, Bengal Native Newspaper Reports 1901, L/R/5/27.

63. *Prabhat*, 01 May 1901, Bengal Native Newspaper Reports 1901, L/R/5/27.

64. *Sanjivani,* 25 April 1901, Bengal Native Newspaper Reports 1901, L/R/R/27.

65. George Curzon, Lord Curzon in India, Thomas Raleigh (ed.), 11 February 1905, p. 497.

66. Mahmud Husain et al, *History of the Freedom Movement: Being the Story of Muslim Struggle for the freedom of Hind-Pakistan, 1707–1947*, (New Delhi: Renaissance Publishing House, 1957), p. 20.

67. Marquess of Crewe, 21 February 1912, Parliamentary Debates: House of Lords, 'The Government of India: Debate on the Recent Changes', Vol. 2, No, 4 (London: His Majesty's Stationery Office, 1912), p. 183, Curzon Papers, Mss Eur F 112/592.

68. For an illustration, see the Native Newspaper Reports: Bombay, IOR L/R/5/160.

69. Ray, 'Communal Attitudes to British Policy: The Case of the Partition of Bengal', p. 37.

70. Khayer Khan Munshi, 'Rajnaitik Andolan o Musulman' Naba Nur, 3rd Yr, 5th No, 1905, in Mustafa Nurul Islam, *Muslim Public Opinion as Reflected in the Bengali Press, 1901–1930*, (Dacca: Bangla Academy, 1973), p. 58.

71. I.H. Qureshi, *The Struggle For Pakistan*, (Karachi: University of Karachi, 1965), p. 27.

72. Gerald N. Barrier, *Punjab Alienation of Land Bill, 1900*, (n.p.: Duke University, 1965), pp. 50–1.

73. Curzon to Hamilton, 21 September 1899, Curzon Papers, Mss Eur F111/158.

74. Barrier, *Punjab Alienation of Land Bill*, p. 57.

75. S.S. Thorburn, *Musalmans and Moneylenders in the Punjab*, (Delhi: Mittal Publications, 1983 [1886]).

76. Gerald N. Barrier, *Punjab Alienation of Land Bill*, and 'The Punjab Government and Communal Politics', in *The Census of British India*, N.G. Barrier (ed.), (New Delhi: Manohar Publications, 1981).

77. David Gilmartin, *Empire and Islam: Punjab and the Making of Pakistan*, (Berkeley: University of California Press, 1988).

78. N.G. Barrier, *Punjab Alienation of Land Bill*, p. 58.

79. Francis Robinson, 'Consultation and Control: The United Provinces Government and its Allies, 1860–1906"', *Modern Asian Studies*, 5:4, (1971): p. 315.

80. Barrier, *Punjab Alienation of Land Bill*, pp. 90–1.

81. Gilmartin, *Empire and Islam*, pp. 28–9.

82. Ibid., p. 27.

83. Ibid., p. 32.

84. Barrier, *Punjab Alienation of Land Bill*, p. 101.

85. Gilmartin, *Empire and Islam*, p. 32.

86. Ibid., p. 34.

87. *Chaudhwin Sadi*, Rawalpindi, 15 January 1900, in Barrier, *Punjab Alienation of Land Bill*, p. 67.

88. Barrier, *Punjab Alienation of Land Bill*, p. 157.

89. *India*, 06 October 1899.

90. *The Tribune* on the ill-feelings generated by the introduction of the Punjab Land Alienation Bill, *Leader*, 9 December 1900 in *Curzon and Congress: Curzonian Policies and the Great Debate*, (Jan. 1899–Mar. 1902), B.L. Grover (ed.), (New Delhi: ICHR and Allied Publishers Limited, 1995), pp. 101–02.

91. Barrier, *Punjab Alienation of Land Bill*, p. 61.

92. *Amritavachani*, 03 November 1900, Madras Native Newspaper Reports, 1899–1900, L/R/5/109.

93. *Vrittanta Patrika*, 15 November 1900, Madras Native Newspaper Reports, 1899–1900, L/R/5/109.

94. *Amritavachani*, 03 November 1900, Madras Native Newspaper Reports, 1899–1900, L/R/5/109.

95. *Rafiq-i-Hind*, 13 February 1900, Punjab Native Newspaper Reports, 1900, IOR L/R/5/184.

96. *Rafiq-i-Hind*, 05 March and 22 March 1900, Punjab Native Newspaper Reports, 1900, IOR L/R/5/184.

97. *Curzon Gazette*, 23 March 1900, Punjab Native Newspaper Reports, 1900, IOR L/R/5/184.

98. *Akhbar-i-'Am*, April 1900, Punjab Native Newspaper Reports, 1900, IOR L/R/5/184.

99. *Rafiq-i-Hind*, 15 September 1900, Punjab Native Newspaper Reports, 1900, IOR L/R/5/184.

100. *Taj-ul-Akhbar*, 29 September 1900, Punjab Native Newspaper Reports, 1900, IOR L/R/5/184. It certainly banished famines, combined with other developmental measures, but it did not end emigration. Barrier contends that it did not eliminate alienation or even debt in the longer term. Barrier, *Punjab Alienation of Land Bill*, p. 84.

101. Barrier, *Punjab Alienation of Land Bill*, p. 73.

102. Nawab Mohammad Hyat Khan on the 'Political Aspect' of the Punjab Land Alienation Bill, 19 October 1900, in *Curzon and Congress*, Grover (ed.), p. 115.

103. Kanwar Harnam Singh on the so-called 'Political Necessity' of the Punjab Land Alienation Bill, 19 October 1900 in *Curzon and Congress*, Grover (ed.), p. 117.

104. Van den Dungen, *The Punjab Tradition: Influence and Authority in Nineteenth Century India*, p. 31.

105. George Curzon, *Lord Curzon in India*, Sir Thomas Raleigh (ed.), p. 173.

106. Barrier, *Punjab Land Alienation Bill, passim.*

107. Gilmartin, *Empire and Islam,* p. 17.

108. Pioneer, The Secret of Lord Curzon's Failure, 19 August 1928, Mss Eur D609/73.

109. *The Tribune,* 25 January 1900, Punjab Native Newspaper Reports, 1900, IORL/R/5/183.

110. *Wafadar,* 22 January 1899, Punjab Native Newspaper Reports, 1900, IOR L/R/5/183.

111. Anil Seal, 'Imperialism and Nationalism in India', *Modern Asian Studies,* 7:3 (1973): p. 326.

112. *Amrita Bazar Patrika*, 22 August 1905, Bengal Native Newspaper Reports, 1905, IOR L/R/5/31.

113. *India*, 25 August 1905.

114. *Hindu Nesan*, 26 August 1905, Madras Native Newspaper Reports, 1905, IOR L/R/5/185.

115. Maconochie, *Life in the Indian Civil Service*, 121–2.

7

The Constraints on the Free Exercise of Viceregal Power

The clamour of the arrogant accuser
Wastes that one hour we needed to make good.
This was foretold of old at our outgoing,
This we accepted who have squandered, knowing,
The strength and glory of our reputations,
At the day's need, as it were dross, to guard
The tender and new-delicate foundations. . . .

Rudyard Kipling, *The Pro-Consuls*

Curzon's Indian Viceroyalty, as noted, has attained legendary status; his towering personality easily lends itself to biographic studies, often verging on the hagiographic in the case of his many admirers and contemporaries, of the 'Great Man' school of historiography. Yet, as this book, *Curzon and the Limits of Viceregal Power: India, 1899-1905,* states, neither Curzon nor any other Viceroy in the colonies ever functioned as autonomous kings in their realms. The Viceroy was not a figurehead; rather, in India he was 'located in an interconnected network of people whose careers were also spent in carving Britain's imperial interests,'[1] incorporating varying levels of authority and power. The structure of colonial governance was not peopled by like-minded officials striving for a common aim.

As the book has progressed, the ways in which Curzon's potential, seemingly limitless at the outset of his Viceroyalty, and bolstered by the factors identified, was constrained by the realities of the networks of colonial governance, have been made manifest. Most of Curzon's actions brought about counter-reactions from his colleagues, who had views and motives that differed from his. As was pointed out in Chapter One, Curzon's exercise of Viceregal authority to achieve his stated ends for Indian administration was aided considerably by some of his colleagues. But if friends in high places were an asset, it is equally evident from Chapter Seven that other equally highly placed friends were in fact responsible for the acrimony that was the hallmark of the later stages of Curzon's time in office. This is just one illustration of the ways in which the structure of power surrounding Curzon operated to suffocate his autonomy of action and reduced his impact on Indian administration. Curzon's efforts to impose his will on the Indian administrative machine, to give it strong leadership, were tempered by wider political, social and economic constraints.[2] Obviously, some of the very factors which served to constrain him had also helped him under certain circumstances and certain points of his term: 'different aspects of the personal equation will condition the individual actor's *potential* effectiveness in different leadership situations.'[3] As always there are extrinsic and intrinsic factors; ones that stemmed from Curzon's own handling of the situation as he analysed it, and ones that he had relatively less control over—people's reactions to him.

Curzon's Temperament: Curzon's own lack of people skills led him to get into snarls with his governors and other officials and they then complained about him to London, with the result that he received rather less cooperation than he would otherwise have got. In this case the policy of permitting the Presidency Governors to correspond directly with London worked to Curzon's disadvantage, especially in the early days of his term, when Havelock was in office at Madras. Of course, that they wrote about their wrongs at the hands of Curzon was not something that could have been forecasted. As Burns notes in his seminal work, 'leaders . . . are cognitive, fact-gathering, calculating creatures who link their goals—and even subordinate them—to the realities of the structures of political opportunity.'[4] Curzon was definitely a fact-gathering and cognitive individual, but he could not dissimulate and sublimate his goals to the extant climate; rather, the extant climate, if it hindered the achievement of his goals, had to be worked around. Curzon could not, or would not, perceive the necessity of biding his time before springing any action upon his colleagues. When he did try to do so, notably over the creation of the NWFP, it resulted in the concerned party being more than usually offended. Obviously, when it came to matters of administration, it did not really matter, as he was the Viceroy and as long as he was able to produce concrete justification for a move, it was usually accepted by the rest of the Government of India. But this lack of a sense of timing and diplomacy let him down in the political realm, especially in his relations with London. Kitchener knew how to pace himself—he was willing to bide his time until Curzon served out a second term to put his plans for Army reform into operation. This Curzon did not know how to do.

Of course, this was tied in to other aspects of Curzon's personality. The fact that he was obsessed by the worry that he would not have enough time to complete his work in India also suggests that he did not think he would be able to hand over power to a suitable successor. He does not seem to have made any attempt at grooming a potential successor, or discussing one with the India Office, at least during his very affable relationship with George Hamilton. The most he did was express horror that Brodrick, or Kitchener, might succeed him. Nor did he appear to think that any potential successor could run India properly; his remark about Kitchener just waiting for him to depart shows that he did not think anyone else capable of controlling India.[5] Obviously this was a power vacuum, one created through omission? Of course, Curzon was merely following historical precedent; there was no tradition of grooming one's successor for the Indian Viceroyalty. Curzon may have observed how the process of choosing a governor for a province almost operated automatically[6] but the process of choosing a Viceroy seems to have been deliberately lackadaisical by contrast. There was no convention even of choosing a Viceroy who belonged to the party in power in England. But the lack of continuity coupled with the fact that the incumbent Viceroy was not usually involved in the choosing of his successor, ensured that policies could be undone at the end of five years by the expedient of choosing a more complaisant Viceroy.

Curzon's abrasiveness has been cited, both by contemporary observers and later historians, as a key reason why he alienated people and could not create a loyalist clique. But there is not much evidence to support this charge: Ampthill, Northcote, Hamilton, Ibbetson, and Mary—self-professed admirers—all suffered his cutting sarcasm and remained, or became, supporters of his policies. In the opinion of this historian, Curzon himself rightly identified the factors that alienated people—his insistence on action. It is possible that the bureaucracy would have put up with his outbursts had they not been accompanied by spot checks on the state of the various projects he insisted they work on. This not only upset them, but made them feel he was straying out of his sphere and infringing their autonomy of action by taking away effective control of their various departments from them. It is significant that Curzon confided his troubles over the recalcitrant bureaucracy solely to Lawrence, who also advocated the above viewpoint.

Excessive Championing of Indian Affairs: While Curzon's obsession with streamlining Indian administration aroused irritation in India, his excessive championing of Indian affairs caused more serious political problems at Home, especially in three quarters; the British Cabinet, the Conservative Party, and the India Office. As observed throughout this thesis, Imperial and Indian interests, and the interests of their respective administrators, were often at variance with the other. Attempting to reconcile both, because this was his self-professed justification for being in India, laid Curzon open to charges of ignoring both British interests, trade, which were the *raison d'etre* for Britain's presence in India and the larger, imperial, interests, of which India, according to London, formed only a proportion. Given that Britain's enormous investments in India were expected to benefit—or at least aggrandise—the English, one cannot really fault Whitehall for their line. Curzon could, of course, have argued that fair play would ensure that Indians would not end up disenchanted with the British presence, which would enable the objective of prolonging their rule in India. The primary reason Curzon's championing of India ran into trouble was his justification for it—he talked about the fairness (or otherwise) of a particular line of policy to the Government of India—as in the case of them paying for the South African war—which was supposed, according to London, to be an agency acting in tandem with it to further British interests in India, not to represent India. But the Government of India could not under any circumstances be said to represent *India*. Had Curzon argued that his proposals were best for Great Britain, or Great Britain's imperial interests, they would not have been so difficult to comprehend in Whitehall. Not that his enthusiasm for securing a better deal for India was well-received in India either. In 1899, he compelled the Sultan of Muscat, despite reservations in London, to annul a concession made to the French, which had given them the right to establish a coaling depot there. *India* scathingly reviewed the case Curzon made out to London:

> Mr Curzon . . . used the common dialect of Jingoism. '*We* subsidise its [Muscat's] ruler. *We* dictate its policy.' When did Mr Curzon become an Indian? What *we* do is to make the poverty-stricken tax payer of India give the Sultan of Muscat a subsidy of £40 000 a year, in order that *we* may add to the dominions of British India. . . .[7]

In a sense Curzon and his sense of fair play and natural justice can be said to have been hampered by his race and background. Contemporary nationalist Indians, an umbrella term which may be used to include persons of varying ideological persuasion, did not greatly question the benefits or otherwise of British presence; it was something they took for granted. But like Curzon, they wanted a better deal for India. Their concerns, even when not addressed, were seen as legitimate on account of their ethnic identities. Curzon's were not because of *his* ethnic identity.

In any case, championing Indian interests against British and/or Imperial interests did not convince his detractors, because his encyclopaedic knowledge of Indian affairs did not necessarily mean he knew as much about other kinds of politics. It may be said that Curzon's very expertise went against him; he possessed what may be said to be 'expert power', derived from his specialist, but stand-alone knowledge of India—it did not further that he was just as knowledgeable about the web of Empire and domestic polity. As Raven and French's seminal study notes, expert power is 'restricted to cognitive systems—in Curzon's case, India—'the expert is seen as having superior knowledge or ability in very specific areas, and his power (or the acknowledgement of it) will be limited to these areas, though some 'halo effect' might occur . . . the attempted exertion of expert power outside the range of expert power will reduce that expert power.'[8] Thus, Curzon was perceived by Balfour, Brodrick, and Godley as a monomaniac incapable of taking a more integrated, all-round view of state policy. And this caused them to examine his Indian legislation, too, with much more circumspection than they otherwise might have, fearing the impact it would have on the frontiers.

Curzon's championing of India had a wider ramification than the India–England tussle. There were imperial aspects to this debate. Events happening in the rest of the Empire—the Gulf, the White Dominions, the Straits Settlements—also worked their influence on Curzon's India. In 1903, Curzon considered abandoning his plans for an English furlough because his acting-Viceroy designate, Lord Northcote, accepted the post of Governor General of Australia, which meant that he could not take over. He continued in part with the Viceregal office after his return, in spite of its 'having become a burden', because the only—in his eyes—worthy successor, the Earl of Selborne, chose instead to succeed Milner in South Africa. This could be described as a leadership crisis. Beyond the poaching of pro-consuls, imperial constraints extended to the realm of domestic politics. Curzon's argument that India was rather more important than any other space occupied by the British was an observation that failed to take into account the growing importance of the ballot box, with the ever-widening enfranchisement of England; they did not always agree with Curzon's notion that England's greatness was built upon her foreign possessions and that the securing of those should be any government's primary priority.

The Conservative Party and Domestic Politics: As noted above, both Hamilton and Brodrick protested when they felt Curzon was placing Indian interests above British or imperial ones; but their protests were limited to the realms of state politics. For the Conservative party, Curzon's Indian policies hurt where it counted the most—at the ballot box. This would appear to be paradoxical, given that Curzon's views about Empire were those normally ascribed to dyed-in-the-wool Tories. But as noted by Niall Ferguson, the Empire was not something that concerned the large mass of the British public. In a reflection of modern-day concerns over outsourcing and off-shoring jobs, Curzon's decisions to impose a duty on cotton imports from Britain angered the Lancashire cotton lobby, and, by extension, the local politicians. After all, the primary theory advanced for Britain's continued presence in India was that India afforded a market for Britain's industrial surplus. The Conservative party naturally felt that Indian interests should ultimately be subsumed to those of Empire. This feeling was all the more enhanced in the opening years of the twentieth century as the Conservative party had one eye on the polls due to the then political instability, itself one of the factors that militated against Curzon. This illustrates how imperial and domestic concerns intermingled and converged within the confines of the political world.

The respective merits of Lancashire vs. Ahmedabad cotton did not disrupt Curzon's Viceroyalty, though it raised questions about his championing of India over Britain. The Viceroyalty thus became an issue linked to British politics, which justified increasing surveillance by the British Government over the Government of India. A more direct and significant way in which domestic politics altered the course of Curzon's Viceroyalty was the resignation of the free-trader George Hamilton, and the subsequent elevation of St. John Brodrick to Secretary of State for India. It is thus possible to trace a long line of events that contributed to Curzon's ultimate resignation.

India Office: The India Office, with the Permanent Under-Secretary for India and—after 1903—the Secretary of State for India, were the most visible and influential factors in curbing Curzon's power. This is perfectly understandable because the Secretary of State, at least, was Curzon's constitutional chief, and Arthur Godley's long entrenchment as the Under-Secretary gave him a hold over every incoming Secretary of State—and possibly led him to regard every incoming Viceroy as merely a transient tenant. The individual roles of both Godley and Hamilton have been discussed in Chapter Two. What is also of importance is how they themselves were affected by the atmosphere in the India Office at large. For example, it is noted in Chapter Two that Hamilton was obliged to weigh Parliament's reactions before assenting to any of Curzon's schemes, as he was terrified of an inquiry into the India Office. Similarly, while Godley has been held to have enjoyed unfettered freedom within the India Office by Kaminsky,[9] the same historian contradicts that notion while demonstrating how Godley's differences with the 'centralizing' Morley drove him to tender an offer of resignation.[10]

The Council of India's rejections of many of Curzon's proposals also had ramifications beyond any one piece of legislation. As noted, the rejections in themselves were not of the type to ruin the defining themes of any Viceroyalty, the Council happily passing major acts such as the Partition of Bengal and the Punjab Land Alienation Act. But Curzon's protests at having the redevelopment of the Viceregal gardens blocked, damaged his stock with Whitehall precisely because it was such a relatively unimportant matter. His differences with the Council also found their way into the press.

But the India Office did not function as a check on Curzon's power solely because of the presence of one Under-Secretary (however permanent) with a will-to-power beyond the confines of his office and one Secretary of State desperate to prove himself. As Galbraith notes, 'the modern state unites within its structure all three sources of power: the political personality, property in the form of the resources it commands and dispenses, and organisation.'[11] In the case of India, the political personality was held to be missing by those in London—they sought to vest it in themselves. By this logic Curzon was reduced to the status of a functionary, part of the 'resources commanded' and held limited power of his own. The India Office seemed to think that 'the creation and maintenance of collective resources is vastly more significant than the distribution of individual resources in determining the structure of power in a society.'[12]

And as can be noted above, the structure and tenor of the India Office did not take shape in isolation. It was influenced by events in the wider political sphere, and these, conflated, served to present unique situations to the Viceroy in India. The office of the Secretary of State became irksome to Curzon only after Brodrick assumed the post; but he did so because the above-mentioned events brought about Hamilton's resignation. And had it not been for Balfour's predilection for filling the government with old friends, Brodrick might not have been in the list of contenders for the post. And then again, even Brodrick's critics have taken the view that he would not have been quite so eager to stamp his authority on the Indian administration were he not desperate to redeem himself after the War Office. Thus, events happening in one part of the political sphere might in themselves have posed problems for Curzon, but when worked into an inter-linked chain of office, they combined to create a situation where it was unsurprising that Curzon should feel that every man's hand was against him. The problem of course lay in the isolation, and yet, connectedness of India. Given that London was the capital of the British Empire, the various strands of information merged and coalesced there into mutually influential patterns, to be used by those administrators based in London for running the Empire as a coherent whole. The advent of the telegraph, its feasibility coinciding with Curzon's Viceroyalty, meant that the Viceroy of India could thus be told what to do as soon as relevant information became available. Sitting in India with the mail two weeks away, it was just not possible for an Indian colonial administrator to command the same kind of information. While links between the various colonies may have been much stronger than has been allowed by most historians, barring a few exceptions,[13] most political information still passed *via* London, in part because the colonies did not have a common aim in terms of foreign policy. Only where the administrators were known to each other, as in the case of Curzon and Charles Hardinge (later, Viceroy of India, 1910–1916) in Persia, could there be exchange of information between two colonial capitals along the same lines as information flowed between London and the colonial capitals. This disjuncture put Curzon at a disadvantage when it came to negotiating with London. He could not use information from beyond India to leverage his justification for any stand he might care to take. This was all the more pronounced in a colony like India, where metropole-periphery connections were much more limited than in the white dominions.

Also, as seen in the case of St. John Brodrick, the mechanics of the India Office and the other departments of the British Government were interrelated, which put further pressure on any incumbent to reconcile various disparate interests. For Curzon to insist that any given Indian interest take priority was merely interpreted as a lack of pan-Empire vision by the India Office, not commendable enthusiasm. For instance, Curzon's objections to India having to bear the costs of the Boer War did not suggest he was a dedicated Viceroy and thus raise him in the estimation of the Secretary of State; it only put Hamilton in the delicate position of having to negotiate a compromise between the War Office and Curzon. Curzon always protested violently at such moments that he merely had India's best interests at heart, and was not after personal glory, but this fact had never been in dispute among the mandarins in London: it was because of his avowed dedication to Indian affairs that he had been appointed Viceroy. What he needed to do after the appointment was integrate the running of Indian administration with the various departments in London—and this is precisely what he appears to have been reluctant to do—whether this stand served India better or not is out of the scope of this book. It is possible that, in fact, the A.J. Balfour-led Cabinet Curzon served under was beginning to shift away from the view that the Empire should be the paramount concern of British politicians, and towards the view that the domestic ballot box should replace it. And the India Office increasingly worked in tandem with the rest of the British Government. In addition, what Curzon saw as the India Office's deliberately putting obstacles in his path might have arisen from a genuine concern to prevent local autonomy from evolving to a degree where it would be difficult to check the running of India from London, which would have made governance under a Viceroy less efficient than himself problematic.[14] And, essentially, for contemporary policy-makers, the purpose of imperial power was stable economic ascendancy. This 'dictated that the Indian empire was meant to be indivisible. Hence, it was ruled through a chain of command stretching from London . . . to India . . . the control of the *Raj* as a system of profit and power had to lie in London.'[15] Curzon's wishing to alter the strength of particular links went against the grain of official imperial thought at the time; Chapter Two illustrated the extent to which Curzon's personal links helped him override the official trend, but his solitary will failed to hold sway once his lone supporter, George Hamilton, resigned office, and he was unable to convince his new superior.

Compliant/Cooperative Colleagues: As the sections above have largely made the point that Curzon's failure to forge harmonious relationships with a large part of the official population kept him from optimising his influence over them, it may appear incongruous to state that forming mutually appreciative relationships also worked to his detriment, but this was indeed the case. The obvious argument to support this is that appreciation of Curzon's qualities blinded his colleagues to his weak spots, as was the case with his wife. But a more significant effect was that loyalist sentiments were taken in London to be evidence of Curzon's authoritarianism, because they seemed to fly in the face of the accepted convention that Curzon was difficult to get along with. Chapter Five has illustrated how Ampthill's 'pro-Curzon' stance was received by the

India Office, and cost him the succession to the Viceroyalty (and therefore a possible chance for Curzon to see his stance on the military issue triumph). This was only one of many such instances. It was a standard complaint from Godley and Brodrick that Curzon's Council was much too complaisant to his wishes: the assumption was that he domineered over them. Not only did this impression make Brodrick and Godley inclined to disparage the credibility of the Council, but it also provided further proof for their contention that Curzon ran the administration much too high-handedly, and cowed his Council into agreement by coercive methods. This in turn heightened their attempts to curb what influence they thought he possessed. They can hardly be faulted. The lack of dissent may indicate complaisance, sycophancy, (which does not bolster the credibility of the alleged sycophant) or the overwhelming presence of an authoritarian boss, the latter being Balfour and Brodrick's assessment.

This turn of affairs, obviously, also rendered unhelpful those elements who would have done the most to support Curzon. It would seem paradoxical that they were unhelpful precisely because they never showed any dissent, but that was indeed the case. And finally, as noticed in Chapter Five, Curzon's supporters were just not as committed—or numerous—as, say, Kitchener's or Balfour's. His Council, for example, held by Brodrick to be his sycophants, did not actually resign over the Kitchener affair after protesting to the Viceroy that they would, if he did. At the crucial moment they failed to demonstrate their support, even though, as Curzon said, he believed himself to have possessed their united adherence.[16] It may be hazarded that they tended toward indifference over issues which the Viceroy might be passionate about. For example, they initially opposed Ampthill when he opposed Kitchener over the military reforms, and then swung round to back him. Paradoxically, it must also be emphasised that by not putting up opposition over major legislation, they were helpful, even if only in a negative way. But the fact remains that he failed to engage with his Council, certainly he did not engage with it to the extent he did with some of his Governors. In addition, the fact that some of his most vocal supporters did not possess political suavity worked against him. A case in point is that of Lovat Fraser, a contemporary editor of *The Times of India* and author of the hagiographic 1911 work *India Under Curzon and After*.[17] Fraser was a keen Curzonian who even ran an anti-Minto campaign in the *Times*, but its—and the monograph's—emphasis on Curzon as a solitary, wronged genius only served to support the modern historian's critique that the Viceroy was incapable of building a team, apart from attracting unfavourable attention from the Balfour–Brodrick camp.

All this, again, may have had something to do with Curzon's early life. While the friendships he formed at school and university certainly carried over into his adult life, he does not seem to have made much effort to cultivate them in a political context. His one political mentor was the ageing Salisbury; he was not part of the governing clique of Balfour's cabinet. This may have been because he did not feel the need to lobby for domestic positions of power, as he devoted his youth to that part of his career which lay outside Britain.

Paradoxically, those colleagues who actually had differing views from the Viceroy, for example, Mackworth Young, did not really affect public perception, or the actual course, of Curzon's Viceroyalty. It was true that Mackworth Young ran a series of vilifying articles in the *Times* against Curzon after they both resigned, but in the meantime much more damage was being done by Francis Younghusband extolling Curzon's virtues to a puzzled Brodrick, who seems to have come to the conclusion that Curzon was trying to build up an influential coterie. This was in part because Curzon's followers tended to be largely those with the same worldview as himself, or those who shared certain similarities. He could not be said to have surrounded himself with a coterie, but many of his associates in India were friends from pre-Viceregal days; Younghusband and Lawrence in particular. Or those he befriended occupied marginal or anomalous positions in the power structure, such as the Home Rule advocate MacDonnell, Northcote in Australia (where he became dissociated from Indian affairs), Ampthill whose comparative youth did put him at a disadvantage in terms of making connections and forging relationships, and Hamilton. With the exception of Hamilton, they were all his official subordinates as well. On the other hand, the people he ended up alienating *were* the power structure: Balfour, Brodrick, Godley, Lee-Warner. This might suggest that Curzon was innocent of realpolitik and did not know how to pick and choose his allies and enemies. As a matter of fact he had relatively little political or administrative experience when he was appointed Viceroy. He had been Under-Secretary for Indian affairs. By contrast, Elgin had been Treasurer of the Household and First Commissioner of Works under Gladstone, as well as Convener of the Fife County Council (this much derided office would, in actual fact, have given him some experience in dealing with dissenting colleagues who had dissimilar views over any questions) and Lansdowne (and later, Minto) had come out to India straight from the Governor Generalship of Canada. Admittedly, Curzon was younger than either of the two when appointed, but a great part of his career had been spent in solitary wanderings, from which he emerged only to unveil a universally lauded tome. This was hardly the setting to inculcate the qualities requisite for a good head of government, required to constantly deal with queries from many different officials each day. It must be remembered that Curzon's compatriot Cromer, with whom he is almost always (and unfavourably) compared, was trained in colonial administration by his cousin Lord Northbrook, in India. In any case, English political reaction to Curzon's appointment was that of alarm— his past explorations did not engender a sense of security in those who had to hand over the administration of India to him. His classics, *Russia in Central Asia* and *Persia and the Persian Question*,[18] published during his pre-Viceregal travels, had the effect of alerting his then acquaintances and the British governing elite (which two bodies were much the same) as to the direction his Viceroyalty's foreign policy could take, especially since the stated aim of his travels was to be a fit Viceroy for India. It is possible that the British Cabinet was reluctant to endorse his plans without extensive scrutiny precisely because they were formed after extensive personal experience and therefore liable to be, if not prejudiced, subjective. The appointment of Francis Younghusband (whom Curzon had struck up a friendship with during his 1894 trek through the Pamirs) to the mission to Tibet in 1904, and Curzon and Younghusband's subsequent vocal support of each other did indeed appear to vindicate the India Office's apparent view that Curzon, if given total autonomy, tended to appoint his own men to ensure that things were done his own way, and assiduously shield them from official censure thereafter. Of course, this could be alleged only in the realm of frontier policy as Curzon had minimal acquaintance with internal Indian administration prior to assuming office; and in fact, his grumbling over the appointment of an old friend to the Bombay governorship should have negated any suspicions that he tended to favour rubber-stamp appointments, but such was not the case.

But, while systems in London converged and commingled to produce a set of circumstances that pretty much controlled the options available to an Indian Viceroy, they were not the only factors which acted as barriers to Curzon having his own way over administrative issues. It is true that because London was the source of all power, the perception of Curzon in London was vital to shaping perceptions of him elsewhere; however, there were also issues within the Indian domestic set-up that contributed to this.

The Communal Equation in India: Even the fiercest critics of the 'partition' of Bengal concede that, as a purely administrative move, it was eminently pragmatic. The move only soured when its communal implications became clear. Thus, it may be inferred that already tense inter-communal relations in India caused unnecessary debate about Curzon's actions. It did not prevent him from doing what he wanted by way of palliative action, but the aftermath was always nastier than it should have been. It will therefore be illustrative to quote a long passage from a review in the Natal Witness of the second volume of Lord Ronaldshay's authorised biography of Curzon, by the Hon. S.V. Srinivasa

Sastri. Sastri notes that in the case of the Partition of Bengal, wherein, according to the author,

> the main motive was the erection of a Muhammadan province to serve as a counterpoise. Your inveterate Tory is a firm believer in the Divide and Rule Policy and when driven to it, is ready to acknowledge his belief and even parade it. . . . Since the Curzonian regime many another costly blunder has been committed under the influence of the policy and *before the full consequences of the parliamentary vote are realised and the national leaders of the people come into their own,* the bureaucracy is bound to err again and again in defence of the citadel. . . .[19]

If the British began to be perceived as the political equivalent of communal rabble rousers, the natural corollary for nationalistic Indians would be to want to get rid of them. Curzon's territorial redistribution was perceived as perpetuating an *extant* division, which impelled the nationalists to protest and damaged his credibility in the eyes of the Indians who had previously lauded him as an exemplary Viceroy. When he resigned, it was bruited about in the *bazaars* of Bengal that he had done so because of censure from Whitehall over his 'partition'.[20] Indian outrage legitimised the efforts of his successors to stamp out 'Curzonization', with full approval from the India Office, because they could argue that the Indians themselves did not want such and such a measure, and it would thus inflame public opinion to press ahead with it.

Consciously, Curzon never let Indian pubic opinion interfere with what he thought were rightful measures. Nor would he modify legislation solely because of negative feedback from Indians. But this only illustrates how dialogues and struggles for power between various types of Indians (a struggle firmly subordinated to, and not normally allowed to participate in the dialogue between the British administrators of India) thrust itself into the relationships of the ruling hierarchy.

Mary Leiter: Historians of the Kitchener affair often quote the Mary—Kitchener correspondence to illustrate Kitchener's duplicity; he wrote affable letters to the Curzons while simultaneously plotting to negate any influence Curzon might possess in London with regard to Army issues. What they overlook, however, is that Mary, who conducted the whole of this correspondence, was taken in by Kitchener's façade. Her attempts to be an unofficial mediator for Curzon did not result in success. Rather, her attempt at boudoir diplomacy backfired heavily, because it caused even Curzon to be deceived about the true nature of Kitchener's intentions. As an aide, Mary was a constraint. As her biographer notes, while the Vicereine did not have any formal role to play in the Indian administration, Mary carved out her own role, taking over social duties and functioning as a liaising agent between Curzon and the Conservative big-wigs while in England. As part of the Viceregal team, therefore, she was active, but she was a sycophant, the sort of follower who clouds the true picture from the leader. As noted in Chapter One, she was an asset because her lack of formal office made her approachable, but increasingly, as ill-health and prolonged absence distanced her from the Indian scene, this role seems to have devolved to Lawrence. Further, different spheres, Indian and British governing circles, did not often overlap, so Mary's Simla charm offensive might not have won her any points among the governing elite back in England. It is also possible that Mary over-estimated the amount of confidences she might generate from Curzon's colleagues; she openly acknowledged her pride at filling a high position in the Empire, and by default, possibly expected people to like her because she was the *Viceroy's wife*. Mary's role is an ambiguity not yet resolved by her biographers. Generally, comments on Mary are curious productions, emphasising on the one hand how little influence she was allowed to have on 'George's will' and on the other how much she fanned his political sensitivity while in London in 1901 and 1904, which one would suppose to be impossible if 'George' really did not listen to her opinions.[21]

It is thus difficult to identify and isolate any one set of factors as having acted as limiting agents to Curzon's drive for a one-man overhaul of the Indian administration. The single-minded dedication towards acquiring encyclopaedic knowledge of Indian affairs that propelled him to the Viceregal office was impeded by a nebulous haze of systemic flaws and checks, the changing dynamics of the balance of power between the rulers and the ruled, and inter-personal relationships re-contextualised from the club to the Cabinet.

Notes

1. Nicola J. Thomas, 'Mary Curzon: "American Queen of India"', in *Colonial Lives Across the British Empire: Imperial Careering in the Long Nineteenth Century*, David Lambert and Allan Lester (eds.), (Cambridge: Cambridge University Press, 2006), p. 307.
2. Cerny,'The Process of Personal Leadership', p. 132.
3. Ibid., p. 132. Italics in the original.
4. James MacGregor Burns, *Leadership*, (New York: Harper Torchbooks, 1979), p. 119.
5. Curzon to Hamilton, 14 May 1903, Curzon Papers, Mss Eur F111/162.
6. See Chapter Four, p. 177.
7. *India*, 10 March 1899, British Library Newspaper Collection, M9211.
8. John R.P. French, Jr., and Bertram Raven, 'The Bases of Social Power', in *Studies in Social Power*, Dorwin Cartwright (ed.), (Ann Arbor: University of Michigan Press, 1959), p. 164.
9. Kaminsky, *India Office*, p. 232.
10. Ibid., 77–81.
11. Galbraith, *Anatomy of Power*, p. 145.
12. D.H. Wrong, *Power*, p. 144.
13. Laidlaw, *Colonial Connections*, p. 14; and Ballantyne, *Orientalism and Race: Aryanism in the British Empire*, pp. 1–3, 9.
14. D.B. Swinfen, *Imperial Control of Colonial Legislation, 1813–1865: A Study of British Policy towards Colonial Legislative Powers*, (Oxford: Clarendon Press, 1970), pp. 3–4.
15. Anil Seal, 'Imperialism and Nationalism in India', *Modern Asian Studies* 7:3, (1973), pp. 326–7.
16. Curzon to Viceroy's Council, 20 August 1905, Curzon Papers, Mss Eur F111/211.
17. Lovat Fraser, *India Under Curzon and After*, (London: William Heinemann, 1911).
18. George Curzon, *Persia and the Persian Question*, (London: Longmans, Green & Co., 1892).
19. 'Lord Curzon: A Great Viceroy', *Natal Witness*, 11 August 1928. Mss Eur D609/73. Italics mine.
20. Cf. Chapter 5, p. 191. The attempt—by both British governmental and popular Indian parties—to attribute Curzon's resignation to the furore over passing

legislation not accepted by the people is also an attempt to deny him legitimacy as a head of government, as it implies an inability to either be convinced by popular opinion, or persuade it to swing in his favour.

21. See Nicolson, *Mary Curzon*. The tone is echoed by Gilmour.

Conclusion

The aim of this book was twofold: to explore and highlight the unused depths of the Curzon Papers and thus to put a new interpretation to Curzon's time in India, exploring the degree of autonomy he managed or chose to exercise in India. This was achieved by taking into account theories of corporate leadership, management and the exercise of power. The book has been an ideological counterpoint to the increasingly patronising analyses of colonial governance and colonial administrators favoured by historians today, in that it takes for granted that Curzon's Indian Viceroyalty was, as such, a good thing. Methodologically, it is also a throwback to the times when the private papers, diaries and correspondence of proconsuls made up the primary source material for studies of their terms in office. This approach holds particular relevance for this book, which examines inter-personal relationships between different individuals in the British Government of India, as many of them stuck to personal correspondence to express their unvarnished views on any given subject. Imperial historians have latterly highlighted the prominent role that the personal connection played in colonial networks of power and influence, governance, and authority. In the case of the Curzon Viceroyalty, the book utilises the private papers from angles hitherto unexamined. Contemporary biographers like David Gilmour do utilise the private papers, but usually only to provide anecdotal evidence and amusing vignettes. I have, instead, by focusing on the private papers, constructed my analyses of inter-personal relationships in the Government of India using the issues the protagonists themselves felt were important enough to warrant personal com-munication. In fact, while Curzon's relationships—or lack thereof—with people have always been a central yet unelaborated theme in biographies. Frictional relationships have been singled out as the root cause of the failure of the Viceroyalty by more than one biographer. But with the exception of the breaking of Curzon's lifelong acquaintance with Brodrick, the course of these relationships has not been charted.

The central conclusion of this book is that Curzon's personal relationships with the rest of the Government of India determined his actions and consequently the outcome of many a legislative move. The first and the last chapters set the boundaries—and in some cases, demonstrated the fluidity of the boundaries—of the camps with which Curzon interacted and negotiated with. These themes were reiterated and developed further in Chapters Two, Three, and Four. Chapter Two further explored the effect of Curzon's lobbying skills—previously dismissed as being too heavy-handed to be effective—and showed how undercurrents between individuals affected Curzon and how Curzon in office (i.e., the fact of him being there) affected individuals' relations with each other. For example, Godley was constrained by Hamilton, as long as he (Hamilton) was in office, from expressing his dislike of Curzon. That a need was felt to develop a counter-weapon to Curzon's influence in India itself, demonstrates, in the opinion of this book, that Curzon was not quite so inept at persuasion and negotiation as has previously been hypobooked. Chapters Two, Three, and Four also showed that just because an individual was pro-Curzon, or even the sort of administrator he approved of in theory, they did not necessarily make his Viceroyalty easier. This is most starkly evident in the case of Mary, as discussed in Chapter Seven, and is also a theme reflected in Chapter Five; Curzon's supporters did not possess the same degree of subtlety his detractors did, a lack most evident in Francis Younghusband's enthusiastic, if rash and counterproductive, campaign in defence of Curzon in the *Times* after his resignation.

The perception of the inter-personal relationship between two individuals as interpreted by a third party, often determined their reactions to, and attempted manoeuvring of, those individuals. This was reflected in the core theme of the book: centre-provincial and inter-departmental relationships. The book endeavoured to advance the subject through its in-depth examination of the centre-presidency relationships (between an individual province and the centre) from angles hitherto unexamined i.e., the individual level, and demonstrating how this relationship was used by those involved, and by the Government of India, to have a bearing on pan-Indian governance. Following on from this, Chapters Two, Three, and Five explored another aspect of the Curzon Viceroyalty for the first time, the process and manner in which Lord Ampthill became a consensual locum, and highlights Ampthill's role in supporting Curzon's line against London, but for which it is entirely possible that the Kitchener affair would have come to a head much earlier than the summer of 1905. It is also important to note that to date Ampthill's role in the Kitchener affair has not been analysed by any historian. The emphasis has always been on Curzon's conduct while in England, but this was largely informed by what he knew his locum to be doing in India. This in turn emphasises how much of Curzon's reactions were informed through collaboration and discussion with his fellow administrators, an aspect of his administration denied by most historians. But as the book shows, collaboration, and not just with Lawrence, was one of the strong points of Curzon's Viceroyalty. In the case of the Punjab Land Alienation Act, for example, his views about the most appropriate legislation evolved as he worked in conjunction with Charles Rivaz. In order to pass legislation, he managed to persuade the then Secretary of State, George Hamilton, not only to accept his methods, but also seek out ways to ensure the passage of the bills concerned through the Council of India. That he was unable to replicate this with Brodrick does not negate his earlier achievement, one which had frustrated Elgin, who had been unable to put through the creation of the NWFP and the Punjab Land Alienation Act in part because of his inability to convince Hamilton. Chapter Six also demonstrated how he worked to co-opt Indian opinion for the above move, thus making the point that Curzon did in fact think it necessary to engage with Indians when political expediency called for it, and, more importantly, could do so to achieve the outcome he desired.

Thus one of the major contentions of this book is that much of what has been written about Curzon's Viceroyalty, and the shape and form of popular and government networks of the time, takes its tone from the later stages of his term of office. Chapter Six demonstrated most starkly how hindsight tends to reify events and distort historical assessments; Indians, right up to the close of Curzon's term, were really quite appreciative of him and certainly did not have a nationally homogeneous opinion about him or about colonial rule. Curzon's ability to elicit diverse opinions, not just in a static fashion but evolving in response to the acts he undertook, among the people he interacted with, most notably the Council of India, and also the Indians, is discussed in Chapters Two and Six, a theme that has been hitherto overlooked by historians who often present the results of his engagement with people at only a single point in time.

* * *

The fact that when, in 1905, Curzon sent in his resignation as Viceroy, the Indian press did not unanimously attribute it to the Kitchener affair, is a testament to how far removed the high (and sneaky) backstairs politics practised in the India Office were from the processes of Indian administration that the full story of the Kitchener affair never became commonplace knowledge until Kitchener's policy collapsed in the Great War. That is not to suggest that the administration of India was carried out by the ICS, the provincial governors and Curzon colluding in rosy harmony; but there were two very distinct streams of power, administrative and political, flowing through the India Office and the Government of India. Curzon, being a parliamentarian, as opposed to a career colonial administrator, attempted, with a remarkable degree of success, to fuse these two in his persona, and succeeded to a remarkable degree before finally failing to overcome growing opposition from an increasingly insecure Cabinet.

By examining these hitherto unexplored themes, the book looked at what may be termed the underbelly of the Viceroyalty; the unexplored counterpoint to the conventional portrait of Curzon as an individual possessing too much hubris. While the book has shown that Curzon in fact collaborated extensively with other administrators to give his Viceroyalty the particular shape it took, his famed self-reliance was not without justification; a great many of Curzon's achievements in India were the result of individual attention and perseverance in the face of official indifference: the establishment of the Archaeological Survey of India being one such. Many more were the result of tackling bureaucratic impasses that had frustrated his predecessors, which involved engaging with various experts with differing views, for instance, the creation of the NWFP, the Punjab Land Alienation Act, and the Partition of Bengal. In one form or another, these reforms exist as he made them, despite multiple changes of government.

This book has thus demonstrated that the Curzon Viceroyalty was neither ineffectual nor authoritarian. It has explained, using evidence gleaned from the writings of his contemporaries, that Curzon was not a bad negotiator, nor a poor team player. Because of his dual identity, as demonstrated throughout the book, Curzon had *two* goals; reinforcing the Empire *and* overhauling the Indian administration, the latter helping to achieve the former goal. Presenting an integrated version of these two different bodies used to pursuing one ideal, required, as the book demonstrates, a skilled networker. Having occupied multiple spheres of political life, he possessed the awareness to criticise and challenge the contradiction of being expected to be, simultaneously, 'independent colonial autocrat and the metropole government's puppet.'[1] Even this binary, being a juxtaposition derived with reference to the imperial metropole, does not cover the 'complexity of colonial relations *in situ*,'[2] where, as the preceding chapters demonstrated, the differing situational circumstances of the many different people in different offices Curzon came into contact with, necessarily affected their reactions to him, and therefore the degree of success he had in engaging with them (even supposing that his very approaches to different issues and persons possessed a degree of sameness). Thus this book also negates the reading that Curzon was an autocrat who did not have the influence he sought precisely because of his autocracy; the individual's own identity in isolation is not always responsible for determining his influence over others.

Curzon's Indian Viceroyalty, therefore, offers a fascinating study as to how one man sought to revitalise the ideal of Empire through the strength of his ideas and his determined efforts to superimpose them upon the administration of the premier Crown possession. What he attempted to do, was, definitely, a do-able task.[3] As noted above, whether he succeeded is immaterial, because the Indian Empire no longer endures. But in late Victorian Britain, given a government stripped of extra-Indian concerns, Curzon's Viceroyalty stands out as the most concerted attempt to wield together a cohesive Empire. Had the situational settings in India and England been different, he might have attained the status Cromer did in Egypt.[4]

From this it may be concluded that Curzon's influence on India, and the degree of power he exercised there, cannot be weighed in isolation, or solely on the strength of his personal traits. It should not be a series of examining multiple but individual strands from the web of relationships that surrounded the Viceroy of India. Rather, as this book has done, it should be an examination of 'multiple meanings, projects, material practices, performances, and experiences of colonial relations'[5] and how these reflect the nature of the personal and official relationships forged between the principal actors. Curzon is widely supposed, even by his contemporaries, to have assumed the Viceroyalty in an era of transition; 'he came at a period when the old order was changing,'[6] but what must be assessed is how much his time in office contributed to that transition, taking the Viceroyalty of India from being a romantic, exotic, colonial posting to an appointment deeply influenced by the English political scene, that also had a bearing on that same political scene. In negotiating for administrative autonomy, Curzon was instrumental in making manifest the ways by which English and Indian politics were irretrievably linked together and the consequent scope and restrictions afforded an Indian proconsul.

Notes

1. Zoe Laidlaw, *Colonial Connections*, p. 62.
2. Antoinette Burton, *At the Heart of Empire: Indians and the Colonial Encounter in Late-Victorian Britain*, (Berkeley: University of California Press, 1998), p. 23.
3. Sir Penderel Moon, *The British Conquest & Dominion of India*, (London: Duckworth, 1989), p. 943.
4. But he did not want to, in fact, become a 'permanent proconsul'. The Empire for him was not a romantic *Boy's Own* field of adventure, but bound by cords to England.
5. Lambert and Lester, *Colonial Lives Across the British Empire*, p. 8.
6. Maconochie, *Life in the Indian Civil Service*, pp. 121–2.

Bibliography

Primary Sources

Ampthill Papers, Mss Eur E233.
Balfour Papers, British Library Manuscripts Collection.
Barnes Papers, Bodleian Library.
Curzon Papers, Mss Eur F111 and 112
Elgin Papers, Mss Eur F84.
Erle Richards Papers, Mss Eur F122.
Hamilton Papers, Mss Eur F123.
Harcourt Butler Papers, Mss Eur F116.
Havelock Papers, Mss Eur D699.
Kilbracken Papers, Mss Eur F102.
Kitchener-Marker Papers, British Library Manuscripts Collection.
Lamington Papers, Mss Eur B159.
Lawrence Papers, Mss Eur F143.
Lee-Warner Papers, Mss Eur F92.
Lyall Papers, Mss Eur F132.
MacDonnell Papers, Bodleian Library.
Midleton Papers, Add Mss 50072–50077, British Library Manuscripts Collection.
Morley Papers, Mss Eur D573.

Private Papers (located at the British Library unless otherwise stated)

Ritchie Papers, Mss Eur C342.
Younghusband Papers, Mss Eur F197.

India Office Records

Minutes of the Council of India, IOR, British Library.
Native Newspaper Reports, IOR L/R/5, British Library.
Proceedings of the Punjab Government, IOR/P, British Library.
Proceedings of the Bombay Government, IOR/B, British Library.

Newspapers at the British Library Newspaper Collection

India, 1898–1905
Paisa Akhbar, 1898–1905.
The Times of India, 1898–1905.

Internet Sources

Oxford Dictionary of National Biography, available from www.oxforddnb.com

Secondary Sources: Books, Theses, and Articles

Adams, Richard and Fogelson, Raymond, eds. *The Anthropology of Power: Ethnographic Studies from Asia, Oceania and the New World.* (London: Academic Press, 1977).

An Indian Mahomedan. *British India from Queen Elizabeth to Lord Reading.* (London: Issac Pilman, 1926).

Bandyopadhyay, Premansukumar. *Indian Famine & Agrarian Problems: A Policy Study on the Administration of Lord George Hamilton, Secretary of State for India, 1895–1903.* (Calcutta: Star Publications, 1987).

Ballantyne, Tony. *Orientalism and Race: Aryanism in the British Empire.* (Basingstoke: Palgrave, 2002).

Ballhatchet, Kenneth. *Race, Sex and Class Under the Raj: Imperial Attitudes & Policies and their Critics, 1793–1905.* (London: Weidenfeld & Nicolson, 1980).

Barnes, Barry. *The Nature of Power.* (Urbana: University of Illinois Press, 1988).

Barrier, N.G. & Crane, Robert I. eds. *British Imperial Policy in India and Sri Lanka, 1858–1912: A Reassessment.* (New Delhi: Heritage Publishers, 1981).

Barrier, N.G. *The Punjab Alienation of Land Bill 1900.* (Duke University Press, 1966.

Bence-Jones, Mark. *Viceroys of India.* (London: Constable, 1982).

Bell, R. *et al,* eds. *Official Power: A Reader.* (London: Collier-Macmillan, 1969).

Bennett G.H. and Gibson, Marion. *Later Life of Lord Curzon of Kedleston, Aristocrat, Writer, Politician, Statesman: An Experiment in Political Biography.* (New York: Edwin Mellen Press, 2000).

Bond, George and Gilliam, Angels eds., *Social Construction of the Past: Representation as Power.* (Routledge: London, 1994).

Brooke, Michael Z. *Centralization and Autonomy: A Study in Organisation Behaviour.* (London: Holt, Rinehart & Winston, 1984).

Brown, Judith M. 'Imperial Facade: Some Constraints upon and Contradictions in the British Position in India, 1919–1935'. *Transactions of the Royal Historical Society*, 5:26 (1976): 35–52.

Burton, Antoinette. *At the Heart of Empire: Indians and the Colonial Encounter in Late-Victorian Britain*. (Berkeley: University of California Press, 1998).

Cannadine, David. *Ornamentalism: How the British Saw Their Empire*. (London: Allen Lane/The Penguin Press, 2001).

Carrington, Michael. 'Empire and Authority: Curzon, Collisons, Character and the Raj'. (PhD Thesis, Coventry University, 2004).

Cartwright, Dorwin, ed. *Studies in Social Power*. (Ann Arbor: University of Michigan, 1959).

Cell, John W. *British Colonial Administration in the Mid-Nineteenth Century: The Policy-Making Process*. (New Haven, London: Yale University Press, 1970).

Churchill, Winston S. *Great Contemporaries*. (London: Leo Cooper, 1990 [1932]).

Clegg, Stewart. *Power, Rule and Domination*. (London: Routledge & Kegan Paul, 1975).

Cohen, Stephen. 'Issue, Role and Personality: The Kitchener-Curzon Dispute'. *Comparative Studies in Society and History 10:3* (April 1968): 337–55.

Cohn, Bernard, *Colonialism and its Forms of Knowledge: the British in India*. (Princeton/Chichester: Princeton University Press, 1996).

Coleman, Bruce. *Conservatives and Conservatism in Nineteenth Century Britain*. (London: Edward Arnold, 1988).

Cook, Scott B. 'The Irish Raj: Social Origins and Careers of Irishmen in the Indian Civil Service, 1855-1914'. *Journal of Social History*, 20: 3 (Spring, 1987): 507–29.

Copland, Ian. 'The Bombay Political Service, 1863–1929'. (D.Phil Thesis, University of Oxford, 1969).

Copland, Ian. *The British Raj and the Indian Princes: Paramountcy in Western India, 1858-1930*. (Bombay: Orient Longman, 1982).

Curzon, George. *British Government in India: The Story of the Viceroys and Government Houses*, Vol. 2. (London: Cassell & Co., 1925).

Curzon, George (edited by King, Peter). *A Viceroy's India: Leaves from a Viceroy's Notebook*. (London: Sidgwick & Jackson, 1984).

Curzon, Grace. *Reminiscences*. (London: Hutchinson, 1955).

Curzon, Mary Victoria (edited by John Bradley). *Lady Curzon's India: Letters of a Vicereine.* (London: Weidenfeld and Nicolson, 1985).

Dahl, Robert. *Who Governs? Democracy and Power in an American City.* (New Haven: Yale University Press, 1961).

Das, M.N. *India Under Morley and Minto: Politics behind Revolution, Repression and Reforms.* (London: George Allen & Unwin 1964).

Davies, C.C. *The Problems of the North-West frontier 1890–1908, With a Survey of Policy since 1849.* (Cambridge: Cambridge University Press, 1932).

Davis, Richard W. 'We are all Americans Now! Anglo-American Marriages in the Later Nineteenth Century'. *Proceedings of the American Philosophical Society*, 135:2 (1991): 140–99.

Dilks, David. *Curzon in India, Vols. 1 and 2.* (London: Rupert Hart Davis, 1969).

Dowding, Keith. *Power.* (Buckingham: Open University Press, 1996).

———, *Rational Choice and Political Power.* (Aldershot: Edward Elgar, 1991).

Durand, Sir Mortimer. *Life of the Right Hon. Sir Alfred Comyn Lyall.* (Edinburgh/London: William Blackwood & Sons, 1913).

Edwardes, Michael. *High Noon of the Raj: India Under Curzon.* (London: Eyre & Spottiswoode, 1965).

Elton, G.R. *The Practice of History.* (London: Fontana Press, 1967).

Evans, Richard J. *In Defence of History.* (London: Granta Books, 1997).

Foucault, Michel (edited by C. Godard). *Selected Interviews.* (Brighton: Harvester, 1980).

Francis, Mark. *Governors & Settlers: Images of Authority in the British Colonies, 1820-60.* (Basingstoke: Macmillan, 1992).

Fraser, Lovat. *India under Curzon and After.* (London: William Heinemann, 1911).

Friedrich, C. *Constitutional Government and Democracy.* (New York: W.W. Norton, 1941).

Fulbrook, Mary. *Historical Theory.* (London: Routledge, 2002).

Galbraith, John Kenneth. *Anatomy of Power.* (London: Hamish Hamilton, 1984).

Gilmour, David. *Curzon: Imperial Statesman.* (London: John Murray, 1994).

Godley, Arthur. *Reminiscences of Lord Kilbracken.* (London: Macmillan and Co., 1931).

Gopal, S. *British Policy in India, 1858-1905.* (Cambridge: Cambridge University Press, 1965).

Goradia, Nayana. *Curzon: Last of the British Mughals.* (Delhi: Oxford University Press, 1993).

Guha, Ranajit. *Dominance Without Hegemony: History and Power in Colonial India.* (Cambridge, Mass.: Harvard University Press, 1997).

Gupta, Amit Kumar. *Between a Tory and a Liberal: Bombay under Sir James Fergusson, 1880-1885.* (Calcutta: K.P. Bagchi and Co., 1978).

Hamilton, Lord George Francis. *Parliamentary Reminiscences and Reflections 1886-1906.* (London: John Murray, 1922).

Hardy, Peter. *The Muslims of British India.* (Cambridge: Cambridge University Press, 1972).

Heffer, Simon. *Power and Place: The Political Consequences of King Edward VII.* (London: Phoenix, 1999).

Hindes, Barry. *Discourses of Power: From Hobbes to Foucault.* (Oxford: Blackwell, 1996).

Johnson, Gordon. *Provincial Politics and Indian Nationalism: Bombay and the Indian National Congress, 1880 to 1915.* (Cambridge: Cambridge University Press, 1973).

Judd, Denis. *Balfour and the British Empire: A Study in Imperial Evolution 1874-1932.* (London: Macmillan, 1968).

Judd, Denis. *Empire: The British Imperial Experience from 1765 to the Present.* (London: HarperCollins, 1996).

Kaminsky, Arnold. *The India Office 1880-1910.* (London: Mansell Publishing, 1986).

Khan, Syed Sirdar Ali. *Lord Curzon's Administration of India: What he Promised, What he Performed.* (Bombay: Times Press, 1905).

King, Peter. *The Viceroy's Fall: How Kitchener Destroyed Curzon.* (London: Sidgwick and Jackson, 1986).

Kochen, Manfred and Deutsch, Karl W. *Decentralization: Towards a Rational Theory.* (Cambridge, Mass.,/Konigstein: Gunn & Hain/Verlag Anton Hain, 1980).

Laidlaw, Zoe. *Colonial Connections.* (Manchester: Manchester University Press, 2005).

Lambert, David, and Allan Lester (eds.). *Colonial Lives Across the British Empire: Imperial Careering in the Long Nineteenth Century.* (Cambridge: Cambridge University Press, 2006).

Lawrence, Walter Roper. *The India We Served.* (London: Cassell and Co., 1928).

Le Maistre, Ian. 'The Second Baron Ampthill's Governorship of Madras and Viceroyalty, December 1900–February 1906'. (MA Thesis, Manchester University, 1977).

Lipsett, H. Caldwell. *Lord Curzon in India, 1898–1903.* (London: R.A. Everett, 1903).

Maconochie, Evan. *Life in the Indian Civil Service.* (London: Chapam and North, 1926).

Magnus, Philip. *Kitchener: Portrait of an Imperialist.* (London: John Murray, 1958).

Martineau, John. *The Life and Correspondence of Sir Bartle Frere, Vol. 1.* (London: John Murray, 1895).

Mason, Philip. *The Men Who Ruled India.* (London: Jonathan Cape, 1985).

Metcalf, Thomas R. *Imperial Connections: India in the Indian Ocean Arena, 1860-1920.* (Berkeley: University of California Press), 2007.

Midleton, William St. John Fremantle Brodrick. *Records and Recollections.* (London: John Murray, 1939).

Mitter, Raj Jogeshur. *Biography of Sir Steuart Bayley, K.C.S.I.* (Calcutta: S.K. Lahiri & Co., 1891).

Moon, Penderel. *The British Conquest and Dominion of India.* (London: Duckworth, 1989).

Moore, Robin. 'Curzon and Indian Reform'. *Modern Asian Studies*, 27: 4 (1993): 719–40.

Morison, Theodore. *Imperial Rule in India.* (London: Archibald Constable and Co, 1899).

Morriss, P. *Power: A Philosophical Analysis.* (Manchester: Manchester University Press, 2002 [1987]).

Mosley, Leonard. *Curzon: End of an Epoch.* (London: Longmans, 1960).

Nicolson, Harold. *Curzon: The Last Phase, 1919–1925: A Study in Post-War Diplomacy.* (London: Constable and Co., 1934).

Nicolson, Nigel. *Mary Curzon.* (London: Weidenfeld and Nicolson, 1977).

Raleigh, Sir Thomas. *Lord Curzon in India: Being a Selection from his Speeches as Viceroy and Governor-General of India, 1898-1905.* (London: Macmillan, 1906).

Ronaldshay, Lord. *The Life of Lord Curzon* (in three volumes), (London: Ernest Benn, 1928).

Robinson, Ronald and Gallagher, John with Denny, Alice. *Africa & the Victorians: The Official Mind of Imperialism*. (London: Macmillan & Co., 1965).

Rose, Kenneth. *Curzon: A Most Superior Person*. (London: Macmillan, 1985).

Roy, Krishna Chandra. *Some Desultory Notes on Lord Curzon's Work in India*. (Calcutta: S.K. Lahiri & Co., 1902).

Sarkar, Sumit. *Modern India, 1885-1947*. (Basingstoke: Macmillan, 1989).

Sayeed, Khalid bin. *Pakistan: The Formative Phase*. (Karachi: Oxford University Press, 1968).

Seal, Anil. *The Emergence of Indian Nationalism: Competition and Collaboration in the Later Nineteenth Century*. (Cambridge: Cambridge University Press, 1968).

Seal, Anil. 'Imperialism and Nationalism in India'. *Modern Asian Studies, 7: 3* (1973): 321-47.

Sharma, A.P. *India's External Relations Under Lord Curzon, 1899-1905*. (9 Ranchi: Subodh Granthmala Karyalaya, 1978).

Sharma, Pramila. *Curzon-nama: Autocrat Curzon, Unconquerable India*. Translated from Hindi by Anjula Bedi. (Bombay: Eeshwar, 1999).

Spangenberg, Bradford. 'The Problem of Recruitment for the Indian Civil Service during the Late Nineteenth Century'. *The Journal of Asian Studies*, 30:2, (Feb. 1971): 341-60.

Stein, Burton, ed. *The Making of Agrarian Policy in British India 1770-1900*. (Delhi: Oxford University Press, 1992).

Swinfen, D.B. *Imperial Control of Colonial Legislation, 1813-1865: A Study of British Policy towards Colonial Legislative Powers*. (Oxford: Clarendon Press, 1970).

Swinson, Arthur. *North-West Frontier: People & Events, 1839-1947*. (London: Hutchinson & Co. Ltd., 1967).

Talcherkar H.A. *Lord Curzon in Indian Caricature*. (Bombay: Babajee Sakharam & Co., 1902).

Thompson, Andrew S. *Imperial Britain: The Empire in British Politics, c. 1880-1932*. (Harlow: Pearson Education, 2000).

Thorburn, S.S. *Musalmans and Moneylenders in the Punjab*. (Delhi: Mittal Publications, 1983 [1886]).

Tinker, Hugh. *Viceroy: Curzon to Mountbatten*. (Karachi: Oxford University Press, 1997).

Twenty-Eight Years in India [C.J. O'Donnell]. *The Failure of Lord Curzon: An Open Letter to the Earl of Roseberry*. (London: T. Fisher Unwin, 1903).

Tyagi, M.S. *British Administrative Policy in India: June 1895-September 1903*. (Delhi: S.S. Publishers, 1982).

Van den Dungen, P.H.M. *The Punjab Tradition: Influence and Authority in Nineteenth-Century India*. (London: George Allen & Unwin, 1972).

Washbrook, D.A. *The Emergence of Provincial Politics: The Madras Presidency, 1870-1920*. (Cambridge: Cambridge University Press, 1976).

Weber, Max (edited by S.N. Eisenstadt). *On Charisma and Institution Building*. (Chicago: University of Chicago Press, 1968).

White, Hayden. *The Content of the Form: Narrative Discourse and Historical Representation*. (Baltimore: John Hopkins University Press, 1990).

Wijeyewardene, Gehan, ed. *Leadership and Authority: A Symposium* (Singapore: University of Malaya Press, 1968).

Williams, Donovan. 'The Council of India and the Relationship between the Home and Supreme Governments, 1858-1870'. *The English Historical Review*, 81: 318, (Jan. 1966): 56–73.

Wolpert, Stanley. *Morley and India 1906-1910*. (Berkeley and Los Angeles: University of California Press, 1967).

Wrong, D.H. *Power*. (Oxford: Basil Blackwell, 1979).

Young, Kenneth. *Arthur John Balfour: The Happy Life of the Politician, Prime Minister, Statesman and Philosopher, 1848-1930*. (London: G. Bell & Sons, 1963).

Wilson, Catherine Mary. 'Sir Walter Lawrence and India, 1879-1918'. (PhD thesis, North London Polytechnic University, 1991).

Index